IF YOU BELIEVE YOU ARE A BINGE EATER,
YOU NO LONGER HAVE TO SUFFER IN SILENCE.
YOU ARE NOT ALONE!

Anne, a 35-year-old graphic designer, learned as a child to keep negative feelings to herself. Instead, she would eat when she felt angry, resentful, and depressed. As an overweight adult, she went on one diet after another and lost weight, but inevitably binged and gained it back.

Alex, 35, saw foods as either "acceptable" or "forbidden." As a result, he was either starving himself on liquid diets or binge eating. One cookie became a binge because he'd been "bad," and guilt and self-blame caused him to lose confidence in his ability to get back in control.

Elizabeth, 50, had spent her life pleasing others. She had grown up as "the good girl," always trying to please her perfectionist parents. As an adult, people took advantage of her nature to the point that she was feeling used and abused but couldn't do anything about it—except binge.

The strategies in this book showed these people and many others how to eat sensibly and end their self-destructive cycles. You too can be a . . .

BINGE BREAKER!™

DR. PETER M. MILLER

BINGE BREAKER!

•

Stop Out-of-Control Eating and Lose Weight

WARNER BOOKS

A Time Warner Company

PUBLISHER'S NOTE: The program herein is not intended to replace the services of trained health professionals or be a substitute for medical advice. You are advised to consult with your health care professional with regard to matters relating to your health, and in particular regarding matters that may require diagnosis or medical attention.

MEDICAL CAUTION: The exercise program described in this book involves moderate-paced walking and is designed for overweight individuals who are relatively healthy. If you have special medical problems such as heart trouble, high blood pressure, respiratory problems, or recurrent back pain, check with your physician before starting.

Binge Breaker!™ is a trademark of Peter M. Miller, Ph.D.

Copyright ©1999 by Peter Miller, Ph.D.
All rights reserved.

Warner Books, Inc., 1271 Avenue of the Americas,
New York, NY 10020
Visit our Web site at www.warnerbooks.com
Ⓦ A Time Warner Company

Printed in the United States of America
First Printing: November 1999
10 9 8 7 6 5 4 3 2 1

Library of Congress Cataloging-in-Publication Data

Miller, Peter M. (Peter Michael)
    Binge breaker : stop out-of-control eating and lose weight / Peter
M. Miller.
        p.   cm.
    ISBN 0-446-67441-9
    1. Compulsive eating—Treatment—Popular works.   2. Weight loss—
Popular works.   I. Title.
RC552.C65M539   1999
616.85'26—dc21   99-21150
                                                                              CIP

Book design by Giorgetta Bell McRee

To Gabrielle, my best friend,
always and forever, darlin'

Author's Note

To maintain professional confidentiality, the names of clients serving as case examples in this book have been changed. In some cases I have modified other relevant descriptive characteristics to further respect the privacy of my clients as well as disguise their identities.

Contents

CONTENTS

BINGE
BREAKER!

CHAPTER 1

....

Beyond Overeating

After spending most of her adult life unsuccessfully trying to lose weight, Janet finally found a diet that gave her hope. After a month of dieting, she had lost 12 pounds and her spirits were high.

Then, at 4:15 Tuesday afternoon, self-restraint came to a screeching halt. Janet was home alone feeling bored, tense, and restless. Her day had been stressful and hectic. Her husband was out of town on business and would not be home that evening. She felt very hungry, strongly craving something sweet.

She just *had* to eat something. To keep dietary damage to a minimum she fixed herself an English muffin with nothing on it. She finished it quickly, experiencing little satisfaction. She fixed another, but this time smothered it with strawberry jam. She ate rapidly, feeling driven to eat more. Rummaging around the kitchen, Janet found an opened package of Oreo cookies that her daughter had brought into the house. The package was still about three-quarters full. Almost without thinking she turned on the television, sat down, and proceeded to eat one cookie after another until the package was empty. As she was eating, Janet felt that she was unable to control what or how much she was eating. She felt uncomfortably full.

When the impact of what she had done finally hit her, she experienced an extreme feeling of self-disgust, anger, and guilt. She later described her thoughts and feelings to me in this way:

> I felt totally defeated. I began thinking, "Now I've really blown it. Stupid! Stupid! Stupid! I'll never do it. This happens every time I try to lose weight. What is wrong with me? Who cares anyway? It doesn't really matter. Nothing matters. I'll never be able to lose weight. Things will never change. I'll always be fat."

With that, Janet gave up. She had planned to eat a low-fat, low-calorie frozen meal for dinner but instead she picked up the telephone and ordered a medium pepperoni pizza with extra cheese to be delivered. After she ate the pizza, her mood became even more negative. She felt embarrassed, depressed, and hopeless. She stopped dieting and exercising and over the next three weeks gained back all the weight she had lost.

If Janet's experience sounds familiar, you may be suffering from a newly described eating syndrome known as *binge-eating disorder*, an eating problem that keeps thousands of women and men from successfully losing weight and keeping it off. Recent studies have shown there is a subgroup of overweight individuals who have a serious problem with persistent out-of-control eating. Successful dieting is not possible unless this basic eating problem is overcome.

BINGE-EATING DISORDER: THE DIETER'S DOWNFALL

Even with the best diets available, you may find it difficult to lose weight and impossible to keep it off once the weight is lost. I found this out with the dietary program that I prescribe in my book *The New Hilton Head Metabolism Diet*. Over a million and a half overweight people have followed this popular plan with the majority doing very well. However, some readers complained to me that their temptation to binge eat was too great to allow them to follow low-fat, low-calorie menus consistently.

Over the past 10 years behavioral scientists have begun an intense investigation of people whose periodic out-of-control eating goes beyond simple overeating. The finding of these studies is that as many as 30 percent of people who seek help for weight loss treatment suffer from what has now officially been diagnosed as *binge-eating disorder*—often referred to by its initials, BED. This syndrome is characterized by periodic episodes of compulsive overeating, or out-of-control eating, that severely hampers attempts at successful weight control.

Binge eaters overindulge when they are alone and they typically feel disgusted, depressed, and embarrassed afterward. They eat large amounts of food even when they are not physically hungry. This eating is much more rapid than usual and continues until the binge eater is uncomfortably full.

If you have binge-eating disorder it will keep you from losing weight. While many people with this problem can lose some weight in the short term, it is almost impossible for them to keep the weight from returning. Because of their binge eating they often gain their weight back quite rapidly.

THE EXTENT OF THE PROBLEM

Early information on binge-eating disorder came from large field studies conducted in the early 1990s by Dr. Robert Spitzer and his colleagues at Columbia University. This research group found that while binge-eating disorder is relatively uncommon in the general public (about 2.5 percent), it is very prevalent among overweight individuals seeking help to lose weight.

Prevalence rates increase with the complexity of the problem. For example, about 16 percent of those attending commercial weight-loss programs such as Weight Watchers meet the criteria for binge-eating disorder. More intensive, comprehensive programs conducted by universities, hospitals, and medical schools are found to have a prevalence of 30 percent. Approximately 70 percent of members of Overeaters Anonymous, a self-help group for overweight compulsive eaters, show characteristics of this disorder.

Binge-eating disorder is found in men and women of all ages. It is slightly more common in women than men with about a 3-to-2 female-to-male ratio. Its prevalence is similar in various ethnic groups.

IS BINGE-EATING DISORDER SIMPLY OVEREATING?

Binge-eating disorder is not just eating too much from time to time. This happens to almost everyone. People with binge-eating disorder feel *driven* to eat, as if they cannot stop themselves. During the eating episode they experience a strong sense of being unable to control their behavior. They also feel great psychological distress over this problem but don't know what to do about it. Binge eating is not simply a matter of being weak-willed because physical hunger is rarely involved.

....

IS BINGE-EATING DISORDER A FORM OF BULIMIA?

Just as binge-eating disorder does not describe simple overindulgence of food, neither does it represent an eating disorder as serious as bulimia or anorexia. Bulimia, or more correctly bulimia nervosa, is a severe eating disorder that occurs in *young women of normal weight.* Not only do bulimics overeat but the most important aspect of their diagnosis is that after overeating they engage in purging (forcing themselves to vomit by sticking a finger down their throat), fasting, or excessive laxative use to compensate for their overeating. They do this, in part, because they have a severe body image disturbance that gives them a morbid fear of gaining weight.

In contrast, while people with binge-eating disorder feel upset and guilty after they overeat, they do not usually purge, fast, or use laxatives to excess. In addition, unlike the normal-weight bulimics, people with binge-eating disorder are overweight. Bulimia is primarily a disease of young women while binge-eating disorder affects men and women of all ages.

Anorexia nervosa is a separate eating disorder that involves a total refusal to eat rather than binge eating. However, all of these problems involve a self-concept that is too much related to body image and not focused enough on internal qualities of character.

The main fact for you to know is that binge-eating

disorder is much less severe and complex than bulimia or anorexia even though it is far more widespread. It is also easier to treat, and the success rates with appropriate treatments are high.

....

THERE IS HOPE!

While we continue to learn about the problem of binge-eating disorder, we now know enough to help anyone with this syndrome. The most important questions in your mind right now may be, "Do *I* have binge-eating disorder?" and, more important, "If I do have it, what can I do about it?"

In the following chapters, I will explain exactly what this problem involves and give you a test to see if you suffer from it. Once we have this information, I will outline a step-by-step program that can help you.

It *is* possible to overcome binge-eating disorder and free yourself from your dependence on food. Traditional weight-reducing diets will not help because they do not address your binge-eating problem. You've probably already discovered this by repeated failures on diets. What you need is the special behavioral, emotional, and dietary program that I will outline for you.

If you have a binge-eating problem you may be suffering in silence, feeling so embarrassed that you don't know where to turn. I want you to know that you are not alone. Binge eating is a common problem among chronic dieters. Unfortunately, binge-eating disorder not only undermines your attempts at weight loss, but also causes you a great deal of suffering and emotional distress.

There is hope. You *can* overcome this terribly frustrating problem and free yourself from the power of food. Once you accomplish this goal, you will stop feeling guilty, start losing weight, and regain control of your life.

CHAPTER 2

······································

What Is Binge Eating?

While the term "binge eating" is of recent origin, the symptoms of this behavior have been recognized in medical writings for over two thousand years. In ancient works, excessive eating was referred to by the Latin *bulimus* or *bolismus*. Derived from the Greek *bous*, "ox," and *limos*, "hunger," the words referred to a ravenous or animal-like appetite. It was only later that distinctions were made between overeating with and without purging (vomiting).

Hippocrates wrote of binge eating as "sick hunger" as distinguished from ordinary hunger. In 1743, *A Medical Dictionary*, compiled by James in England, described a condition labeled "true boulimus" characterized by intense preoccupation with food and overeating within a very short interval.

Prior to the eighteenth century, binge eating was thought to be caused by any one or a combination of digestive dysfunction, stomach acidity, gastritis, defective gastric secretions, congenital structural abnormalities, brain disease, and head injury. It was only in the nineteenth century that theories regarding the possible psychological nature of this behavior emerged.

Early treatments focused on warming and comforting the stomach both internally and externally. Medieval medical prescriptions for this problem included the consumption of red wine, hot spices, and fatty, greasy foods. Apparently, fatty foods were prescribed to cause intestinal discomfort to discourage further eating. Other early remedies required all food to be boiled to "jelly" prior to eating. Fortunately, our current treatments are less traumatic, more palatable, and certainly more effective.

It was not until the 1950s that Dr. Albert Stunkard, a renowned obesity expert at the University of Pennsylvania School of Medicine, published the first case report of what he labeled "binge-eating syndrome" in *Psychiatric Quarterly*. Actually Dr. Stunkard's patient was responsible for naming the disorder when he compared his episodes of excessive overeating to an alcoholic's binge drinking. The patient was a 37-year-old high school teacher who was 5 feet 9 inches tall and weighed 272 pounds. He had been overweight since childhood. He sought treatment because he was being considered for a position as principal and could not pass the required physical exam because of his weight.

He told Dr. Stunkard that eating had become an obsession with him. He thought about food almost all the time. He spoke of his eating in terms of victories and defeats or instances of "I was good" or "I was bad." Being "bad" meant succumbing to temptation, breaking his diet, or going to great lengths to prevent anyone from witnessing his "shameful" acts of eating. His eating pattern was very erratic with few regularly scheduled meals. He often ate out of frustration with day-to-day stresses.

During one binge, he stopped off at a grocery store on the way home from work and proceeded to buy a cake, several pieces of pie, and cookies. He remembers driving through town with one hand on the steering wheel and the other hand stuffing food in his mouth. He ate rapidly, paying little attention to what or how much he was eating. Afterward, he was totally stuffed and uncomfortable. He felt extremely guilty and upset over his behavior.

Unfortunately, little attention was paid to the binge-eating problems described in this case study for the next two decades. Then, in the 1980s, interest in this problem was renewed with the publication of several important studies. (I am pleased to say that the first of these research papers was published in the international journal *Addictive Behaviors*, of which I am editor in chief.) Throughout the 1990s several major universities and medical schools have launched a concerted effort to find out more about binge eating and its treatment. Based on these studies we now can better define binge eating and the important clinical features associated with it.

....

THE DEFINITION OF A BINGE

Clinically, a binge is defined as eating—within a time period of two hours or less—an amount of food that is definitely larger than most people would eat under similar circumstances. People diagnosed with binge-eating disorder binge two or more times a week.

In defining a binge, the context in which the eating occurs is important. What would be considered excessive consumption at a typical meal might be normal or average during a holiday meal or a special celebration. On the other hand, eating a meal-size portion of food as an in-between-meal snack would be considered excessive.

A single episode of binge eating does not have to be restricted to one setting. Consider the case of Joan. As a veteran dieter who never had been successful at losing weight because of her binge eating, Joan read a magazine article on binge eating and came to me for help. One of her recent episodes of binge eating illustrates the point that this behavior need not be confined to one location.

It was a Saturday and Joan and her husband were scheduled to go to a dinner party that evening. She had gained 30 pounds over the past six months and had been avoiding social engagements out of embarrassment.

At four o'clock in the afternoon she tried on the one dress she knew would still fit her and would also help to hide her extra pounds. Disaster! The dress wouldn't fit! Not even close. She couldn't even zip it up. She felt devastated. "What's the use?" she thought. She was alone in the house since her husband was out playing golf so she went straight for the refrigerator. She took out the ice cream, put a large portion in a bowl, covered it with chocolate sauce, and proceeded to eat it all. After finishing off another large bowl, she felt depressed, guilty, and angry with herself. She not only had "broken" her diet but she would have to go to the party in one of her larger-sized outfits, one that she felt made her look like a "tank."

Once at the party, she overate hors d'oeuvres and even had dessert. She felt self-conscious the entire evening and couldn't relax. Upon returning home, she stayed up later than her husband to watch television. She felt so miserable and embarrassed that she ended up eating a whole bag of chocolate chips that she had bought a few weeks earlier to make cookies.

Joan's overeating had begun in the afternoon, continued at the party, and kept going upon her return home. While this pattern is considered binge eating, frequent snacking on *small* amounts of food throughout the day would not be called bingeing.

LOSS OF CONTROL

The primary clinical feature of binge eating is the experience of *loss of control* over the impulse to eat rather than the absolute amount of food consumed. In fact, a sense of lack of control over the impulse to eat is a mandatory element in the diagnosis of this problem. Loss of control refers to a feeling that one cannot stop eating or control what or how much one is eating.

Indicators of impaired control over impulses to eat include:

- Eating very rapidly
- Eating until feeling uncomfortably full
- Eating to excess when not physically hungry
- Eating alone because of embarrassment
- Feeling disgust, guilt, or depression after overeating

You can feel out of control during a binge even if you planned it. At other times, overeating may be more spontaneous or impulsive, accompanied by a feeling of being "driven to eat." If you feel you are not able to prevent overeating from occurring or if you are no longer controlling your eating because you feel that overeating is inevitable, you have lost control over food.

FEELING "SPACED OUT"

Although not one of the defining features of a binge, some people experience a feeling of being "numb" or "spaced out" during their binges. Eating is not an unconscious act, but mental awareness is clouded. One of my clients described her experience this way:

I was alone at home last night feeling restless, bored, and lonely. I had bought two large, family-sized bags of M&Ms on the way home from work. I know I shouldn't have bought them but I just couldn't help myself. I began to eat one M&M after another, very rapidly. I felt as if I were in a daze. I felt robotic and machine-like. I realized what I was doing but, in some way, I didn't. This probably doesn't make a lot of sense but my mind just stopped working.

You may or may not have had such experiences but if you have, they are related to the loss-of-control sensations that accompany a binge.

THE ANATOMY OF A BINGE

One reason that internal, subjective factors such as feelings of loss of control are so essential to the definition of binge eating is because it is difficult to obtain general agreement on exactly how much food constitutes a binge. Dr. William Johnson and his colleagues at the University of Mississippi Medical Center set out to answer the question of what most people consider to be binge eating. He asked a group of overweight binge eaters to keep detailed written food diaries of what they ate each day. A total of 746 eating episodes were recorded.

The subjects in the study were then asked to judge which of these episodes they would consider to be binges. Dr. Johnson next asked a separate group of people who were neither overweight nor binge eaters to rate the same eating episodes as to whether or not they were binges. Finally, he enlisted the aid of dietitians and asked them to determine which of these eating episodes were binges.

After all the judgments were compared, Dr. Johnson found a high level of agreement between the dietitians' ratings and the ratings of the normal, nonbinge eaters. Both groups tended to rate the same eating episodes as binges. There was little agreement between the judgments of either of these groups with the binge eaters. The binge eaters labeled many more of their eating episodes as binges, even those with less food involved. They were defining a binge more by their feelings of lack of control than by the type or amount of food eaten. These findings show that perceived loss of control (which may vary considerably from person to person) is crucial in defining binge eating.

OBJECTIVE VERSUS SUBJECTIVE BINGES

Studies such as the one just described have led to the classification of binges as being either *objective* or *subjective*. An objective binge is an eating episode that involves an unusually large amount of food (given the circumstances) *and* a feeling of loss of control. In a subjective binge, you perceive the amount of food you are eating to be unusually large but it actually is not, given the circumstances. You do, however, feel out of control. Most people with binge-eating disorder report both types of binges each week, with about half being objective and half subjective. Although subjective binges do not result in as much weight gain as objective ones, they do cause similar guilt and emotional distress.

WHEN AND WHERE PEOPLE BINGE

Although binges can occur at any time of day, people with binge-eating disorder are more likely to have problems with eating in the late afternoon and late evening. The most likely time for a binge is four o'clock in the afternoon.

Late evenings trigger binges especially if you are alone or if everyone else in the family has gone to bed. Depression and other negative emotions become more pronounced in the evening hours and can lead to emotional eating.

In fact, Dr. Albert Stunkard, the psychiatrist who first reported this type of binge eating, has identified a pattern of eating known as *night eating syndrome*. This syndrome is characterized by eating very little or nothing early in the day followed by binge eating in the evening. The pattern is often associated with insomnia. Many people with this problem awaken during the night and binge before going back to bed. Whether this behavior is just a variation of binge-eating disorder or constitutes a separate eating disorder remains to be seen. I believe it to be so typical that it is simply another form of binge-eating disorder.

Binge eating occurs almost exclusively when a person is alone. In fact, the sudden appearance of another person may end the overeating episode. Compulsive overeating can happen anywhere—at home, while driving, or at work. You may notice that certain situations are more associated with your binges than others, such as during the preparation of a meal or just after grocery shopping.

HOW MANY DOUGHNUTS MAKE A BINGE?

How many doughnuts would you have to eat to feel you had binged? This is exactly the question that Drs. Catherine Greeno, Rena Wing, and Marsha Marcus of the University of Pittsburgh Medical School (one of the major centers of research on binge-eating disorder in the United States) asked overweight binge and overweight nonbinge eaters in a recent study. Before I tell you how their research subjects responded, take out a piece of paper and write your own answer to this question. Next, answer the same question for candy bars, cookies, slices of bread, hot dogs, and slices of pizza.

The binge eaters and nonbinge eaters showed a high level of agreement as to what constitutes a binge in most of the food categories. This may be related to the fact that both the binge eaters and nonbinge eaters were all overweight (unlike the control group of non-overweight individuals in Dr. Johnson's study mentioned earlier).

How do your responses compare? Do you agree that approximately 4 doughnuts makes a binge? Perhaps your answer depends on the size or type of doughnut. What about the other categories? The binge eaters said that a binge begins at 3 candy bars, 9 cookies, 5 slices of bread, 3 hot dogs, or 5 pizza slices.

When asked, "What is the typical amount of each food that you eat?" and "What is the most amount of each food that you have ever eaten?" the binge eaters reported eating more than the nonbinge eaters in every category. They typically ate larger amounts of these foods on a regular basis. During their worst binges the average responses for the "most amount eaten" (all at once) categories were: 5 doughnuts, 4 candy bars, 15 cookies, 4 hot dogs, 6½ slices of bread, or 6½ slices of pizza.

....

THE MOST TYPICAL
BINGE FOODS

The doughnut study brings up the subject of what foods are considered binge foods. Since the type of food eaten does not determine a binge, any food can qualify as long as you eat an unusually large amount and experience a sense of loss of control. The following comments from Rose, a 43-year-old attorney from New York City, illustrate this point.

> I can binge on just about anything. In fact, I know when my weight-loss program is in trouble when I begin to eat too much fruit. Whoever thought about bingeing on fruit? In fact, I had a dietitian tell me not to worry because fruit is a healthy choice and the more fruits and vegetables in my diet, the better. However, when I binge on fruit I can eat four or five apples or bananas and feel totally out of control. I'm upset more by the feeling it gives me than by what I'm eating. Once I start to binge on fruit, then cookies, ice cream, and candy bars aren't far behind.

In fact, Rose's fruit binges served as a warning to her that she needed help. They allowed her to take action, to call me for a booster session, before her binge eating spread to high-fat, high-calorie foods and ruined her efforts at losing weight.

Rose's experience is probably not typical since most people with binge-eating disorder binge on high-fat, high-carbohydrate foods. Typically, women have more of a tendency to crave foods that are high in fat and sugar such as cakes, candy, and ice cream. Men seem to crave high-fat, high-protein foods such as steak, cheese, and butter. These gender differences are certainly not absolute and you may find that you crave both categories of foods.

Although many binge eaters feel they are addicted to sugar, they actually consume more fat than carbohydrates in a binge. For example, premium ice cream contains 57 percent of daily values of fat and only 36 percent carbohydrates per serving. Most "sweet" foods contain as much, if not more, fat than sugar. Studies have found that when sugar and fat content in foods are modified without an individual's knowledge, binge eaters eat more of the high-fat-content foods.

Generally speaking, when you eat foods that you perceive as being "forbidden," you are more likely to feel that you have binged, no matter how much you have eaten. Four hundred calories of candy may seem more like a binge to you than the same number of calories of chicken, potatoes, or cottage cheese. However, binge experiences are very personal and individual, as we saw with the case of Rose. We are only beginning to learn about the nature of binges and the thoughts and feelings associated with them.

BINGE CALORIES

In addition to the emotional toll resulting from binge eating, this behavior also leads to the accumulation of large numbers of unwanted calories. Weight loss or weight maintenance becomes impossible.

Studies show that the typical binge of overweight binge eaters includes between 400 and 1,000 calories, although binges of several thousand calories are not unheard of. The overeating episodes of those with binge-eating disorder typically contain fewer calories than the binges of people suffering from bulimia. Bulimics have been known to consume as many as 20,000 calories before they stop eating and counteract the effects of the food by forcing themselves to vomit.

Binge calories add up—fast. Five binges a week at 700 calories per binge adds up to 3,500 calories per week above and beyond the calories in your regular meals. Every time you accumulate an extra 3,500 calories, you will gain a pound on the scale. That's a pound a week, fifty-two pounds in a year just from binge eating.

In addition to extra calories, the discouragement you experience from binges results in on-again, off-again dieting and the accumulation of even more calories. Controlling binge eating is an absolute must for successful weight control.

Now that you know the details of binge-eating disorder, I'm going to give you a test to see if you have this problem.

CHAPTER 3

....

Do You Have Binge-Eating Disorder?

Although we have been studying binge eating in overweight individuals for 20 years, it was only in 1994 that this problem was officially recognized as a specific clinical syndrome. Before I give you a test to see if you suffer from this problem, let's look at how overweight binge eaters differ from overweight people who do not binge. See how many of these characteristics apply to you.

....

EARLY ONSET OF OBESITY

If you are overweight and a binge eater there is a greater likelihood that you have been overweight since you were young. Most people with binge-eating disorder have been overweight since they were teenagers. About two-thirds of binge eaters developed a weight problem before age 18 with the remainder becoming overweight after this age.

Binge eaters have more weight to lose than those who do not binge. They are about 30 pounds more overweight than dieters who do not binge.

....

FREQUENT DIETING

Binge eaters are yo-yo dieters, going on one diet after another, losing weight but always regaining it. Because of binge eating, weight is often gained back very quickly. Binge eating makes dieting extremely difficult, if not impossible. Because of your binge eating you may not last very long on diets.

My clients report a lifetime average of eleven serious attempts at weight loss, all of which have failed. Losing and regaining weight time after time is known as *weight cycling* and can be extremely distressing.

The average total lifetime weight loss for each individual I have treated is 211 pounds. This sounds like an unbelievable figure, but take a moment to add up all the weight you have lost and then regained in your lifetime and you may be surprised by your total.

Mary consulted me after a lifelong battle with her weight and her binge eating. At 50 years of age she had been overweight since college. She gained 25 pounds during her freshman year, and over the years her weight increased to 230 pounds. Over the years she had dieted more than 30 times, losing and regaining over 750 pounds. She had given up hope until she learned that her binge-eating disorder was the reason she could not diet successfully. I am pleased to say that after a course of treatment, as prescribed later on in this book, Mary is doing extremely well. She has lost her weight and only suffers from an occasional "mild" binge.

I don't care how many times you have dieted unsuccessfully. Once you learn to control your binge eating, you'll discover a new sense of personal control that you've never experienced before. Mary is a completely different person with a whole new attitude about herself and her life. She never thought it was possible.

PREOCCUPATION WITH FOOD

Overweight binge eaters think about food and worry about overeating to a much greater extent than overweight nonbinge eaters. Dieting, food, and fears about losing control over impulses to eat are a constant problem. One of the most gratifying results of successful treatment is that you will be free from this obsession.

DISSATISFACTION WITH APPEARANCE

While many overweight people worry about appearance, binge eaters have an intense preoccupation with their bodies. They are very concerned with how overweight they are and think about it often. And as we know, self-worth and self-esteem are very much related to appearance.

Listen to the words of Mark, a 32-year-old sales-man who successfully overcame his binge eating and lost 48 pounds.

When I weighed 233 pounds I felt miserable. I'm not just talking about lack of energy from carrying all that weight around. I actually felt like a different person. I have always felt self-conscious about my weight. I have always hated my body. Looking in the mirror, I would often feel disgusted with myself, ashamed of myself. I have always been aware of my weight, especially in public. It made me feel terribly in-secure. This has been a real problem for me since I'm in sales. I'm sure my weight affected my work.

Now that I've stopped bingeing and lost my weight I feel like a different person. I am much more confident and sure of myself. I give a lot more credit to others than I used to. I have dis-covered positive qualities about myself that I never even thought about before. I realize now that my feelings about myself were too much re-lated to my weight and not what really matters.

Unlike bulimics, people with binge-eating disorder do not have to be overly thin to feel good about themselves. They just want to be at a reasonable weight. However, concerns about weight and shape, particularly when they serve as the basis for your self-esteem, must be addressed as part of the treatment process. (I'll have more to say about this later when we discuss the causes of binge-eating disorder.)

MOOD PROBLEMS

Binge-eating disorder is associated with higher rates of major depression throughout your lifetime. Binge eating becomes worse during these periods of depressed mood. Even without major depression, binges are often triggered by anger, sadness, or anxiety. Other psychological problems associated with binge eating include panic attacks, emotional impulsivity, and the excessive use of alcohol.

THE BED TEST

The following is a test to see if you have binge-eating disorder. One disadvantage of diagnostic tests is that they place people into categories of either having or not having a particular problem. Keep in mind that there are variations of every problem and that your binge-eating syndrome may be severe, moderate, or even mild. Even if you only have some of the symptoms of binge-eating disorder, you may still need help. If your binge eating, no matter how infrequent, keeps you from achieving your weight goal, you need help as much as a more severe binger.

> **IMPORTANT NOTE:** The diagnosis of binge-eating disorder assumes that you do *not* regularly engage in any of the following behaviors. If you do any of these *twice a week or more*, you may be suffering from bulimia nervosa. This problem is more serious than binge-eating disorder and would require an evaluation by a clinic or a professional specializing in eating disorders.

- Make yourself vomit in order to avoid gaining weight after binge eating
- Take more than twice the recommended dose of laxatives in order to avoid gaining weight after binge eating
- Exercise for more than an hour specifically to avoid gaining weight after binge eating
- Take more than twice the recommended dose of diuretics (water pills) in order to avoid gaining weight after binge eating

The BED Test

1. During the past six months, did you often eat, within any two-hour period, what most people would regard as an unusually large amount of food?
   ____Yes   ____No

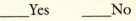

2. When you ate this way, did you often feel you could not stop eating or control what or how much you were eating?

____Yes   ____No

3. During the past six months, how often, on average, did you eat this way—that is, large amounts of food plus feeling that your eating was out of control? (There may have been some weeks when it was not present—just average those in.)

____Less than one day a week

____One day a week

____Two or three days a week

____Four or five days a week

____Nearly every day

4. Did you *usually* have any of the following experiences during these occasions?

- Eating more rapidly than usual?

  ____Yes   ____No

- Eating until you felt uncomfortably full?

  ____Yes   ____No

- Eating large amounts of food when you weren't physically hungry?

  ____Yes   ____No

- Eating alone because you were embarrassed?

  ____Yes   ____No

- Feeling disgusted with yourself, depressed, or guilty after overeating?

  ____Yes   ____No

5. In general, during the past six months, how upset were you by overeating (eating more than you thought was good for you) or by the feeling that you could not stop eating or control how much you were eating?

_____Not at all
_____Slightly
_____Moderately
_____Greatly
_____Extremely

How to Analyze Your BED Test Answers

Question 1—Episodes of Binge Eating

If you have binge-eating disorder you would have answered *Yes* to this question. If you answered *No*, you are saying that you do not experience overeating episodes and, therefore, would not have a binge-eating problem.

Question 2—Loss of Control

People with binge-eating disorder would answer *Yes* to this question regarding feelings of lack of control over the impulse to eat. If you answered *No*, your overeating would not be considered binge eating since loss of control is a defining feature of this problem.

Question 3—Frequency of Binge Eating

The diagnosis of binge-eating disorder requires that you binge, on the average, two or more days a week. If your answer indicates that you binge only one day a week or less, you have a mild to moderate binge problem that is not frequent enough for you to be diagnosed with binge-eating disorder. However, if infrequent binge eating causes you distress or interferes with weight control, you would still benefit from the treatment program I outline in later chapters.

Question 4—Indicators of Loss of Control

This question lists the major indicators of impaired control over the impulse to eat. Marking *Yes* to three or more of these indicators shows that you fall within the binge-eating disorder diagnosis. If you answered *Yes* to only one or two of these, you have a milder binge-eating problem.

Question 5—Your Reaction to Binge Eating

People with binge-eating disorder are *Greatly* to *Extremely* upset by their binges. They can be upset either by the amount of food they eat and the subsequent weight gain caused by it or by their feelings of being unable to control their eating. If you answered by checking either one of these categories, you would be in the binge-eating disorder category. If you answered that you are *Moderately, Slightly,* or

Not at all upset by your binge eating, you might not be facing up to the significance of your problem (especially if all of your other answers indicate binge-eating disorder). It could be that in the total scheme of things in your life, there are other problems that are causing you more stress at the present time. Just remember that you will not be able to deal with your weight problem successfully without overcoming your binge eating.

Please do not think of this as an all-or-nothing test to determine whether you suffer from binge-eating disorder or not. As I have indicated, you may not have all these characteristics, but you may still have a binge problem. Even if your problem is less severe it could still bother you, serve as a major obstacle to weight loss, or become worse.

Now that you know the extent of your binge-eating problem, it's time to examine the factors that caused it.

CHAPTER 4

....

Predisposing Reasons Why You Binge

The answer to the question of what causes binge eating is a complex one. Like many human conditions, binge eating is the result of a variety of factors that interact with one another. We are still learning exactly why some overweight people binge and others do not. Binge eating is caused by the interaction of social, psychological, and biological factors.

I will describe what we know about the development of binge eating and the likely reasons why you might have this problem. Before we talk about what causes specific episodes of binge eating, let's begin with factors that predispose you to overeat in the first place. Certain factors in your background may have made you more susceptible to developing a binge-eating problem. These include: (1) heredity, (2) family interaction patterns, and (3) society's obsession with thinness.

....

GENETICS

It is a well-established fact that heredity determines your body size, shape, and weight. Without genetic influence, if neither of your parents were overweight, your chances of being overweight are about 34 percent. If one parent was overweight, the chances of an infant developing the problem rise to 40 percent. Your chances of being overweight reach 80 percent if both of your parents were overweight. In fact, the majority of overweight binge eaters have been overweight since childhood.

In addition to total body size and weight, heredity determines your shape and body features. You may be very dissatisfied with your body, not because you are overweight but because you inherited a tendency to carry your fat in your thighs, buttocks, or stomach.

For someone who has always been thin, dieting would not be needed, and binge eating would be much less likely. Genetically programmed overweight or body shape predisposes you to dieting. In turn, food deprivation and continual self-restraint predispose you to binge eating. As we shall see later, early-onset overweight causes problems in self-esteem, which also makes binge eating more likely.

Jennifer is a 34-year-old married mother of two who has been overweight since childhood. Her husband is a sales executive with a large firm and she is a pediatric nurse. When she came to me for help with binge eating she reported a history of being in the

99th percentile for weight even from birth. Both of her parents fought weight problems most of their lives. Her mother had been overweight since childhood and in spite of repeated dieting was 60 pounds overweight. Her father was less overweight but the extra 20 pounds he carried around caused his blood pressure to fluctuate in spite of medication.

Jennifer remembers dieting most of her life. She recalls as a child not being able to eat what other children were eating. In fact, she does not remember a time in her life when she was not either restricting her food intake or going to the other extreme and binge eating. Jennifer was obsessed with the fact that she would never be able to lose weight because her body size was inherited. I assured her that this was not the case. Many people who have been overweight since birth are able to manage the problem especially if they overcome their binge eating.

I explained to Jennifer that her compulsive overeating was due, in part, to the fact that she has always had to restrict what she was eating. As I will describe in a moment, the process of chronic dieting changes your biological and psychological makeup in such a way that binge eating becomes very likely.

FAMILY ENVIRONMENT

Family interactions and communication patterns also set the stage for binge-eating problems. This can happen in a variety of ways.

EMPHASIS ON APPEARANCE

In some cases, families place strong emphasis on physical appearance and thinness. Being overweight is viewed as a character flaw and a blight on the entire family. The overweight daughter or son is an embarrassment.

Iris, a 49-year-old school administrator, experienced this pattern throughout her life. Her mother was a slender, attractive woman who had a successful career as a fashion model when she was young. Throughout Iris's life, everyone remarked on her mother's great beauty and slim figure.

From the beginning, Iris took after her father, who was a tall (6 feet 5 inches), massively built man. His large stature had proved to be an asset during his successful football career as an offensive lineman at a large southeastern university. After his college days, he gained weight and had a continual battle with the scale.

Although Iris was tall with large features, she actually was not overweight as a child. She remembers feeling self-conscious about being the largest and tallest child in her classes at school. She especially remembers one incident when she was ten years old. Her father was transferred and the family moved to a new city. When she entered her new fifth-grade classroom, the other students sat quietly and stared at her. She felt extremely embarrassed. Only later did she realize that because of her size, her fellow pupils thought she was the new teacher, not a new student. She was totally mortified.

Iris became even more self-conscious about her appearance because she was so much the opposite of her mother. Since body size and shape had been so important throughout her own life, Iris's mother had always been concerned about her daughter's appearance. She continually urged Iris to diet and would remark, "If only you hadn't taken after your father, you could have been beautiful." She took Iris to doctors only to be told that her daughter was naturally tall and big and nothing needed to be done about it.

Food and weight took on enormous importance between mother and daughter. Iris's mother was always watching what her daughter ate and commenting on it. The only time Iris felt "free" to eat was when she was alone. This led to binge eating beginning in her teenage years. Whenever her mother was not around Iris would binge. Unfortunately, a pattern of binge eating and poor self-esteem continued into her adult years.

OVERPROTECTION

Families who are overprotective with children can also predispose a person to binge eat. In such families, mothers are often overprotective and critical of their daughters. In such an atmosphere, children find it difficult to develop independence and an identity of their own. Autonomy and self-reliance are stifled. Feelings of love are expressed in an immature, babyish way or through food. Negative emotions are usually avoided.

Girls who grow up in these families lack confidence and have poor self-esteem. They suffer from dependency conflicts, in which they strongly desire personal independence but, through insecurity, seek out dependency relationships. They eventually resent their need to be dependent on those close to them.

These conflicts usually result in passive-aggressive behavior typified by passive resistance. Passive resistance is doing the opposite of what someone wants you to do such as a teenager who "forgets" to study for an important exam after being reminded several times by her parents to do so. Since food was important as an emotional salve in childhood, eating can be the focus of this resistance. It's the "I'll show you; I'll eat whatever I want" reaction.

SUPPRESSION OF FEELINGS

Families in which children develop binge-eating problems often unwittingly teach their offspring to suppress the expression of negative emotions. Unpleasant feelings are not discussed. As these emotions build up they are expressed indirectly through compulsive eating, psychosomatic illness, or impulsive behavior.

Anne, a 35-year-old graphic designer, consulted me about a lifelong binge problem. At the time I first saw her she was 5 feet 5 inches tall and weighed 175 pounds. Her binge eating began during adolescence, before she even had a problem with her weight. Her parents were pleasant, caring people who enjoyed their children. (Anne has an older brother and a younger sister.) Her father was a district manager who traveled a great deal. Her mother took pride in taking care of the family especially when it came to food. She kept a well-stocked cupboard, prepared overabundant meals, and baked cakes and cookies almost every week.

Neither of Anne's parents dealt directly with negative feelings. When disagreements arose, her father would quietly escape to his workshed for one of his woodworking projects. Her mother would retire to her room, and when she returned to the kitchen she would bake something. The children were told that it was not right to talk about how you feel. "If you can't say something nice, don't say anything at all," her father would say. Anne remembers that as a small child she became very angry with her mother for not letting her go to a friend's house to spend the night. She stomped her feet and said, "You're not being fair. I don't like you anymore." She was told that she should never say that again, that she should love her mother no matter what, and that something must be wrong with her to even think in such a way. Anne felt guilty for even feeling angry and started to think that there was, indeed, something wrong with her to have such feelings.

She quickly learned to keep her emotions to herself. Because food was so available in the household, Anne would eat whenever she felt angry, resentful, or depressed. Eating not only allowed her to vent her feelings but provided a calming influence that soothed her emotional distress.

Her compulsive overeating occurred frequently enough, especially during adolescence, that she began to gain weight. During high school she gradually developed a significant weight problem that caused her to be very self-conscious and shy. Anne found herself going on one drastic diet after another. She would lose some weight but binge eating always caused her to regain whatever she had lost. Unfortunately, this pattern continued throughout her adult life until I was finally able to help her identify and overcome her compulsive overeating problem. Her treatment program included breaking the connection between emotions and eating and teaching her new ways to deal with anger and resentment.

Not everyone who has these family interaction patterns, the hereditary predisposition to be overweight, or both develops binge-eating problems. These factors simply set the stage for the development of the problem.

SOCIAL ATTITUDES ABOUT THINNESS

Since the 1960s our society has idealized thinness, particularly in women. To be attractive, accomplished, worthwhile, and desirable, women think they must be thin. Studies have shown that 70 percent of adolescent girls feel they are too fat and need to lose weight. One survey of several high schools found that two-thirds of *average-weight* girls were trying to lose weight. Almost 20 percent of girls who were underweight were dieting.

Models, movie stars, and actresses in commercials are, for the most part, very thin. In fact, the average Miss America contestant, supposedly the "ideal" as far as weight and shape are concerned, is 15 percent *underweight*. To put this in perspective, one of the diagnostic criteria for anorexia is a body weight that is 15 percent below a person's desirable weight. What society considers the perfect woman is actually abnormally thin.

In addition to labeling extreme thinness as perfection, society also shuns overweight. Children as young as six years of age describe silhouettes they are shown of overweight children as "lazy," "dirty," "stupid," and "ugly." In comparing photos of average-weight, overweight, and facially disfigured people, young children judge the overweight to be the least likeable.

Studies in the business world have shown that 16 percent of employers would not hire someone who is overweight under any circumstances, regardless of their qualifications. Even health professionals are not immune to this stereotype: one survey found that even physicians view their overweight patients as weak-willed and unattractive. A total of 78 percent of overweight patients say they have been treated disrespectfully by the medical profession because of their weight.

You may have felt these stereotypes throughout your lifetime. Dissatisfaction with your body shape or size can lead to chronic dieting and, as I mentioned previously, dieting can lead to binge eating. This is especially true if your body image is so negative that it adversely affects your self-esteem.

CONCLUSION

Your heredity, family interaction patterns, and society's attitudes about thinness can all set the stage for a binge-eating problem. They don't guarantee that you'll become a binge eater but they increase your susceptibility. Whether or not you develop binge-eating disorder depends on specific psychological and biological factors outlined in the next two chapters.

CHAPTER 5

....

Psychological Reasons Why You Binge

Whether or not you become a compulsive overeater depends on five specific psychological factors. Let's examine each of these to see how they may be contributing to your binge-eating problem.

....

DIETARY RESTRAINT

You probably realize that the experience of restraining your appetite and limiting your intake of food changes the way you think and feel about food. Because of this, dieting can be one of the causes of binge eating.

To your body, dieting and starvation are one and the same. Dieting triggers a "survival response" whereby physical and psychological changes occur to ensure that you *will* eat in order to "save your life."

Did you ever wonder what would happen if someone who is not overweight, who never had a weight problem, was put on a diet? If you have a spouse, sister, or friend who can eat anything and not gain weight, perhaps you've fantasized about this question. They probably have no idea what you are going through.

Back in the late 1940s, a group of researchers at the University of Minnesota did just what you've been thinking about. They put 32 normal-weight, healthy men on a diet for six months to see what would happen. The men were conscientious objectors from military service during World War II who volunteered to live together in a controlled environment for a year. They ate meals prepared in a special dietary kitchen.

During the first three months of the study the men were fed a normal amount of food. For the next six months they were placed on what the researchers called a "semistarvation diet" of 1,600 calories a day. If you are a veteran dieter you may not consider 1,600 calories to be that low but it was low enough for these non-overweight men to lose 25 percent of their body weight.

During the six months of dieting the men experienced dramatic changes. They felt tired and irritable. They lost their ambition and were apathetic about life. They had difficulty concentrating. Many suffered from depression. These symptoms were not present before dieting began.

Not only did the men complain of hunger but they became preoccupied with food. They talked about food and daydreamed about eating. Reading cookbooks became a popular spare-time activity. Several men developed a pattern of binge eating (although they were living in a controlled setting they were able to go out and purchase other food). Some could not adhere to the diet and began to compulsively overeat huge quantities of cookies, ice cream, and candy. They reported feeling out of control and unable to stop eating—a prime characteristic of binge eating.

These men were experiencing the same mental and physical problems that one has when dieting. The lesson to be learned here is that *these experiences are the normal result of dieting.* You may have thought that your preoccupation with food signified a lack of willpower or a deficiency in character strength, but even average-weight people who are put on diets have the same reactions you do. And, for you, dieting may be a way of life rather than a once-in-a-lifetime experience.

During the final three-month phase of the study the men were fed a normal amount of food once again. Most returned to their normal eating patterns and gained back their lost weight. For most, the psychological symptoms of dieting as well as the obsession with eating disappeared. However, some continued to binge eat and to be preoccupied with food. This may also happen to you. Even when you're not dieting, you may still binge, causing weight gain that requires even more dieting. It's a vicious cycle that seems never-ending.

This is not to say that you shouldn't try to lose weight. Antidieting proponents have suggested that you should learn to live with your body size. The fallacy of this argument is that at least 300,000 deaths a year are attributable to being overweight. Obesity, even by a little, increases your risk of diabetes, high blood pressure, heart disease, gallbladder disease, some forms of cancer, and respiratory problems.

Even if you don't have these problems now, the longer you stay overweight, the more likely one or more of these problems will develop. Remember, also, that obesity is a progressive disorder that gets worse with time. The natural course is for you to gain more and more weight as time goes on.

There *is* a way to lose weight and avoid the pitfalls of binge eating. That is what this book is all about. We simply must recognize the natural effects of the body's "survival response" and learn techniques to deal with them.

ALL-OR-NOTHING THINKING

If you are like most binge eaters, you react to life with dichotomous thinking, a tendency to view experiences as either black or white, all or nothing, good or bad. This is especially true with food and eating. You probably think of foods as being either "acceptable" or "forbidden," "legal" or "illegal."

This perfectionistic thinking results in an eating style in which you are either starving yourself or overeating. The word "moderation" is not in your dictionary. All-or-nothing thoughts cause binge eating because once you have broken a dietary rule, you feel you have "blown your diet" and you give up. You convince yourself you have failed and that your willpower has abandoned you.

Alex, a 35-year-old journalist, presents a good example of how all-or-nothing thinking influences binge eating. This is how he described one of his binge-eating episodes to me.

> I was doing okay on my diet until my wife went out of town for the weekend to visit her mother. I was working on a writing assignment and fighting an urgent deadline. I felt rushed and stressed.
>
> I went to the grocery store to buy some coffee. That's all I needed because my wife had prepared low-calorie meals for me to eat while she was gone. Once in the store, I began craving a nice, juicy steak. I love steak. As I passed the meat counter, I couldn't resist. I bought a 16-ounce T-bone steak. Then I figured, "If I'm going to have the steak, I might as well go all the way." So I bought french fries and a six-pack of beer to go with it. I also bought a can of peanuts and a package of cheddar cheese.
>
> All I could think about was eating. Once home, I cooked the steak on the grill and, while cooking, began drinking beer and snacking on the peanuts and cheese. I ate the whole can of peanuts and half the package of cheese. After

that, I finished off the steak, french fries, and the rest of the beer.

When it was all over I felt totally stuffed and uncomfortable. My stomach felt like it was going to explode. I felt miserable and very, very guilty. I thought, "There I go again. Now I really blew it. I've ruined my diet. I'll *never* be able to lose weight. I have absolutely no willpower. Maybe I can get started again next week." After calculating that I had eaten over 4,000 calories, I felt totally dejected and worthless. I gave up and didn't get back on my diet for a month.

Alex's thought pattern after the eating episode is typical of dichotomous thinkers. He views his dieting efforts as all-or-nothing. When he is following all the rules, he is "on" the diet. When he eats anything that is not allowed, he is "off" the diet. Once he breaks a dietary rule, he has crossed over the line and there is no going back. Guilt and self-blame cause him to lose confidence in his ability to get back in control.

All-or-nothing thinking is both a cause and a result of overeating. When faced with a dozen homemade chocolate-chip cookies you may be so tempted that you go off your diet and eat one of them. If you view this as a "relapse" as opposed to a temporary "lapse" in your program, you may abandon your efforts to stay on your diet and finish off the rest of the cookies. You say to yourself, "One cookie is just as bad as a dozen." Common logic would tell us that from a caloric and nutritional standpoint, this is simply not true.

....

MOOD AND PERSONALITY

Most dieters report that binges are most often triggered by emotional distress. You probably realize that you are much more likely to overeat or "go off" your diet when you are angry, resentful, anxious, depressed, or lonely. The more this happens, the more you begin to mislabel emotional distress as "hunger." After a time you simply don't know the difference.

The reason you eat when you're upset is because the act of eating reduces anxiety and has a calming effect. If you've been dieting, eating is even more relaxing because you don't have to struggle to restrain your cravings anymore. In addition to psychological relief from eating, certain foods produce brain chemicals that have a tranquilizing effect on mood. I'll have more to say about this in the next chapter on biological causes of binge eating.

Eating also serves to distract you from stressful emotions. Stressful situations lead to negative thoughts and feelings that are upsetting. We seek escape and relief from distress by narrowing our mental focus away from the upsetting thoughts, focusing instead on food. Binge eating is a mindless, robotic activity during which you are not thinking about anything, including life's problems.

When you are stressed out, food, eating, and

weight seem more manageable and less anxiety producing than the personal problems in your life. All this happens automatically without full-conscious awareness. The end result is that overeating is defined as the "problem" as opposed to the personal issues that caused the stress in the first place. Because of this, you stay locked into your binge-eating pattern and never confront the significant issues in your life.

As you know, emotional relief from eating is short-lived. As eating continues or shortly after it stops, you are plagued by feelings of guilt and discouragement. The stress resulting from a binge causes you to continue bingeing or to give up on yourself and your dieting efforts.

In addition to this stress/food connection, serious bouts of depression are much more prevalent in people with binge-eating disorder. It is not known whether depression is a cause or an effect of binge eating but it can be a significant factor in triggering compulsive overeating.

Betty, a 60-year-old divorced photographer from Boston, suffered from episodes of depression most of her life. Her depression was cyclical, occurring once or twice a year and lasting for several weeks. She had seen a psychiatrist off and on for several years and was taking antidepressant medication. The medication and periodic therapy were helpful, and although her depressive episodes continued, they were less severe.

For the past three years her depression would begin in January and last until spring. Because of this she was diagnosed with Major Depressive Disorder with Seasonal Pattern Specifier (sometimes referred to as Seasonal Affective Disorder). During these times she felt little energy and would sleep for hours on end. She felt sad and worthless and derived little pleasure from anything in life. She intensely craved carbohydrates and would often gain 20 to 30 pounds during the winter season.

Food was the only thing that would give her pleasure and, at least, momentary relief from depression. Her overeating as well as her weight gain made her feel guilty and even more worthless than she already felt.

If you suffer from cycles of depression whether mild or severe, they will interfere with your attempts to control your binge eating. Often, professional treatment for depression must go hand in hand with treatment for binge-eating disorder. Actually, some antidepressant medications have been found to alleviate depression and reduce cravings, especially for sweets.

There is no general personality type that is more prone to binge-eating disorder. However, in addition to depression, overweight individuals with binge difficulties have a higher prevalence of three specific personality problems: dysthymic disorder, panic disorder, and borderline personality disorder. The exact nature of the relationship of these personality disorders and binge eating is not known, but they probably represent a susceptibility to emotional distress resulting in a decrease in impulse control.

If you have dysthymic disorder you suffer from a chronically depressed mood. You have low self-esteem and view yourself as uninteresting and incapable. You have accepted your lot in life and probably think, "That's just how I am." You feel inadequate and have trouble making decisions. You are quick to criticize yourself. You may have chronic sleep problems. You use overeating to obtain pleasure and self-gratification but all it does is make you feel guilty.

People with panic disorder suffer from recurrent and unexpected panic attacks. Panic attacks are characterized by accelerated heart rate, trembling, shortness of breath, sweating, feelings of choking, chest pains, abdominal distress, light-headedness, and fear of losing control or going crazy. Since some of these experiences can also be symptoms of a heart attack, those suffering from panic attacks often wind up in hospital emergency rooms. In fact, when reassured that there is no medical cause for these symptoms, people with panic disorder still fear that the attacks indicate heart trouble or seizure disorder. Panic attacks are so scary because they occur "out of the blue" with no specific triggering event.

If you have a diagnosis of borderline personality disorder, you are a very impulsive person. You act before you think. In addition to binge eating you may also drink too much alcohol, smoke too much, or spend too much money. You are moody, have trouble controlling your emotions, and frequently "fly off the handle." Your temper can be intense and inappropriate. You have an unstable self-image and intensely fear abandonment by others. You may create a self-fulfilling prophesy by being demanding and suspicious of those close to you. You may suffer from chronic feelings of emptiness and binge eat in order to fill this void.

Remember, these conditions require diagnosis and treatment by health professionals. Whether you fall into one of these personality categories or not, you can still overcome your binge-eating problem. However, you may need psychological treatment in order to help you implement your binge-eating program.

SELF-ESTEEM AND BODY IMAGE

As a binge eater you probably have a very low opinion of yourself. Low self-esteem is both a cause and an effect of binge eating. If you have low self-esteem you are extremely self-critical and quick to find fault with yourself. You may try to please everyone and fear that you won't live up to the expectations of your family and friends. When people compliment you, you probably downplay their praise or think they are not being sincere.

You may also be critical of and dissatisfied with your body weight and shape. Most overweight binge eaters cannot remember a time when they were not self-conscious about the way they looked. Some actually view themselves as grotesque.

One way in which body-image problems have

been studied is to ask people a series of forced-choice questions as to whether they would prefer being overweight to having various physical handicaps. When given this choice, most severely overweight individuals say they would rather be deaf, diabetic, or dyslexic. In fact, almost 10 percent said they would rather have a limb amputated than be overweight.

Your mind can make your weight problem seem worse than it actually is. Overweight individuals are three times more likely to overestimate their body size compared to non-overweight people. This is especially true if you have been overweight since childhood.

There are some people who go to the other extreme and view themselves as being much lower in weight than they actually are. These people usually do not weigh themselves, do not want photos taken of themselves, and do not even want to discuss their weight. They are in denial. I weighed a woman once who had convinced herself that she was 45 pounds lighter than she actually was. She had not weighed herself in months and refused to discuss or think about her size.

Over the years, your opinion of yourself becomes closely tied to your body image. You may begin to judge your worth as a person based solely on your body weight. I often ask clients to give me a brief description of themselves so that I can begin to get a better idea of their self-concept. Here are two self-descriptions to illustrate this point.

Description #1

I am a quiet, withdrawn person. I feel ill at ease when I first meet people. I know they are probably looking me over and wondering why I'm so fat. I have very little confidence in myself and always think twice before I express an opinion about anything. I am not a very interesting person. My life is rather dull and boring.

Description #2

I am a reserved, laid-back person but I wouldn't say that I'm shy. I have several close friends that I enjoy very much. I have a good sense of humor and people generally like me. I feel that I have accomplished a great deal in my life and am proud of myself. I am looking forward to taking on new challenges and expanding my horizons over the next few years.

You may be surprised to find out that these two different self-descriptions came from the same person, a 29-year-old computer consultant. During the time of Description #1 she weighed 185 pounds, approximately 45 pounds overweight for her height. Description #2 occurred three months after she had successfully overcome her binge-eating problem and had lost 34 pounds. Once she learned to control her eating and lose weight her view of herself and her life improved dramatically.

It is amazing how a person's body weight becomes so connected to their sense of personal worth. One of the goals of my binge-eating program is to break this connection and to teach you to base your self-esteem on internal qualities of character rather than appearance, body shape, or weight. Concern about your weight is one thing but allowing your body weight to totally determine your mood and self-worth is another.

Overconcern with your body weight can make you so desperate that you seek out drastic, very low-calorie diets. Overly restrictive diets result in such deprivation that binge eating is even more likely. In turn, when you lose control and overeat, your self-esteem worsens, causing you to feel incompetent and ineffective in controlling your weight. Then your concern over your body and anxiety about weight gain intensify.

HEIGHTENED SENSITIVITY
TO FOOD CUES

Contrary to popular belief, hunger is only related to our eating behavior in a small way. In fact, studies show that people who are overweight have a difficult time determining when they are really hungry. Because of your weight, dieting history, and bingeing, your eating has become less related to the internal sensations of hunger and more to external factors such as the availability and appearance of food.

Many years ago, Dr. Albert Stunkard, the weight-control expert mentioned earlier, asked volunteers—

some overweight, some not—to swallow a gastric balloon attached to a tube that was fitted to a measuring device. When the balloon reached the stomach it was inflated with water. Whenever stomach contractions occurred, indicating physical hunger, the measuring device was activated. All volunteers had been without food for approximately 15 hours. Subjects were asked to let Dr. Stunkard know when they felt hungry.

There was a big difference in how the overweight subjects responded to this situation compared to those who were not overweight. When those who were not overweight reported feeling hungry, their stomachs were contracting, showing a real physiological response. With the overweight subjects, there was no relationship between stomach contractions and reports of hunger. When they felt hungry, *nothing* was happening. In fact, sometimes when they reported hunger, stomach contractions were occurring but they were not paying attention to them. Their hunger was more psychological in nature.

What this means is that people who binge are less responsive to internal hunger cues than other people. On the other hand, they are more responsive to external food cues. The appearance of food as well as its smell and taste turns on their appetite. They crave food because it's there. Real hunger is irrelevant.

Heightened sensitivity to external cues increases when you are dieting. This is part of the body's survival response. Your body cannot tell the difference between dieting and starvation. Since the body is so

programmed for survival, it makes dieting more difficult by making you more sensitive to the sights,
smells, and tastes of food. Your body wants you to
pay more attention to food so you will eat and not
starve.

A major part of overcoming binge eating is to
learn what real hunger is and what it feels like. You
must learn to become less sensitive to food and more
sensitive to your internal hunger feelings. I will show
you exactly how to accomplish this goal through my
Mindful-Eating Program.

CHAPTER 6

Biological Reasons
Why You Binge

Brain chemicals and hormones also influence appetite and eating. Let's take a quick look at the biological factors that play a role in your overeating.

THE INSULIN EFFECT

Insulin plays a key role in the regulation of appetite and this role is more pronounced if you are overweight or if you are dieting. Your body transforms carbohydrates you eat into glucose for energy. Insulin, secreted by your pancreas, helps transport glucose throughout your body and unlock the cells so they can utilize it.

When you eat, the production of glucose triggers your pancreas to secrete insulin. However, insulin can also be produced *in anticipation* of eating. In a study at Yale University, Dr. Judith Rodin showed how the pancreas responds to the mere sight of food.

She presented overweight and non-overweight women with appetizing food. They were told to look but not touch.

As they looked at and thought about how appealing the food was, their bodies began to react physically as well as psychologically. Dr. Rodin found that each woman's insulin level began to increase in response to the craving. Remember, insulin output reduces and regulates blood sugar in your blood. Since these women had not actually eaten anything there was no need for their blood glucose to be regulated. The result was that the insulin lowered their normal blood glucose to a below-normal state, a condition known as hypoglycemia. A lowered blood glucose level is associated with hunger—*real, physical hunger.*

Insulin was triggering the appetite and physically driving the women to eat. A psychological craving had been transformed into physical hunger. Insulin can be produced whenever you smell food, prepare a meal, or even think about food.

This insulin reaction, which increases hunger and craving, occurs with greater intensity in people who are overweight and in people who are dieting. Since the body interprets very low-calorie dieting as starvation, the insulin reaction may represent the body's attempt to entice a chronic dieter to eat for survival. The insulin reaction is also due to the repeated association of the sight, smell, and thought of food with binge eating. Because of the frequency of these associations, the binge eater's body becomes conditioned to anticipate food in response to external food cues.

Merely seeing food sets off an anticipatory response that, in the past, only occurred after eating.

This pre-eating insulin response is more pronounced in the overweight because of their heightened sensitivity to the sight and smell of food (mentioned in the previous chapter). This is why one of the main goals of my treatment program is to teach you to become more aware of your internal hunger and less reactive to external food cues.

METABOLISM

When you diet, your metabolism is suppressed because your body interprets dieting as starvation and as a threat to life. By slowing the metabolic rate, your body is trying to save energy in order to keep you alive. The longer you diet the more your metabolism is suppressed. Very low-calorie diets and high-protein diets are especially bad for your metabolism.

Because of this metabolic suppression, binge eating during a diet will cause more of a weight gain than binge eating when you are not dieting. One binge can result in a two- to three-pound weight gain because of the excess calories that are not being burned as well as the water retention caused by rich or salty foods.

A weight gain of this magnitude can have devastating psychological effects, resulting in guilt, discouragement, and depression. If you gain little or no weight from one overeating episode you might be able to handle it and forge ahead. But, if a binge causes you to gain the three pounds you lost last week, you would be very, very discouraged and possibly give up.

I ask some of my clients to keep a written journal of their binge episodes so that we can analyze and understand them. Ken, a 42-year-old engineer, was very motivated to change and kept detailed written records of his binges. He was doing this even before he came to me for help. He would often try to lose weight by using canned formula diet drinks and avoiding food altogether. Without realizing it he was drastically suppressing his metabolism and setting himself up for failure.

The following is a typical entry in his journal:

Friday, April 17, 1998

Today was not a good day for my diet. I have been drinking my diet formula drinks every day for two weeks and trying to avoid high-calorie food. I had a tough day at work because our company had lost an important customer be-cause of a stupid mistake by one of our salespeo-ple. On my way home from the office I was starving. I felt weak and drained. I saw a Krispy Kreme doughnut shop just up ahead and couldn't resist. I ordered a half-dozen chocolate-covered, cream-filled doughnuts at the drive-through window. I could hardly wait to get at them. As I continued driving home, I ate the doughnuts one after another until they were all gone. As I drove into the driveway, I felt miserable. Why did I do it? I couldn't believe how stupid I had been. I even hid the doughnut box so my wife wouldn't find out what I had done.

This incident threw Ken off his diet for the weekend. He felt like a failure and had three more binge episodes on Saturday and one on Sunday. On Monday morning he woke up, determined to do better.

Monday, April 20, 1998

This morning I was ready to get myself back in control. I was not going to let one bad weekend ruin my diet. I had lost weight for the past three weeks and I was feeling proud of myself. I made the mistake of weighing myself first thing in the morning. I couldn't believe it! I had gained four pounds from Friday to Monday. I've never gained so much weight in such a short period of time in my life. This upset and discouraged me so much that I said, "What's the use? I'll never lose weight. It just doesn't matter anymore." I lost all of my enthusiasm for getting back on the diet.

If Ken had not been following such a drastic, low-calorie diet he never would have gained so much in a weekend. His diet, which provided only 600 calories a day, drastically lowered his metabolism so that the weekend of binge eating resulted in a four-pound weight gain and total discouragement.

As I have discussed in my book *The New Hilton Head Metabolism Diet*, there are ways to overcome this metabolic suppression while dieting. I have included these methods in my binge-eating program so that an occasional slip will not have such devastating effects on your weight.

....

SEROTONIN

Binge eating may be driven by a need to increase serotonin, a brain chemical that produces a feeling of relaxed calmness. Serotonin levels increase when we eat carbohydrate foods. That is why, compared to protein or fatty foods, carbohydrates such as pasta, bread, and chocolate have a soothing, mood-altering effect on us.

Some experts feel that we binge on certain foods to increase serotonin to soothe us. That is why you want to eat when you're stressed out. Food becomes your antidepressant or antianxiety medication. It may be that your brain does not produce enough serotonin and you are driven to eat in order to get more. It may also be that you enjoy the mood changes resulting from serotonin more than others.

Jackie, a 46-year-old woman from Atlanta, described her reaction to chocolate in this way:

When I eat candy I feel like a totally different person. It calms me. I feel tranquilized. It's a drowsy, relaxed sensation. My body feels warm and heavy. I hate to admit this, but chocolate gives me a mental and physical pleasure that I don't get from anything else. I feel like a drug addict.

I am sure you have noticed that sweets have a calming, relaxing effect on you. They also make you drowsy and less alert. Have you also noticed that when you eat breakfast (which most overweight people do not eat) you feel drowsy and hungry by late morning? That's not because you ate breakfast but because of what you *had* for breakfast.

Let's suppose you had French toast or pancakes versus yogurt or cereal and milk. A carbohydrate breakfast of French toast or pancakes would raise your serotonin, causing you to feel tranquil but not very alert. If you had a business meeting at 10:30 A.M. you might have trouble staying awake and concentrating. A little more protein for breakfast might be better.

Too much protein and not enough carbohydrates would make it more likely that you will binge. High-protein, low-carbohydrate diets help to cause binge eating because they lead to lowered serotonin levels. Your body will crave carbohydrate foods on these diets in an attempt to increase serotonin.

I mentioned earlier that you may suffer from bouts of depression if you are a compulsive overeater. One theory regarding this relationship is that both depression and binge eating are related to serotonin. Depressed people have low levels of serotonin, and some antidepressant medications (Prozac and Zoloft, for example) work by increasing serotonin levels.

Preliminary evidence suggests that these medications may also help with binge eating but, unfortunately, their effects may only last for a few weeks.

Finally, many women report that just prior to their menstrual cycle they experience strong cravings to binge, especially on sweets. Women who suffer from PMS have less serotonin during this time, which may explain their strong cravings. In fact, premenstrual women eat 30 percent more carbohydrates than they do at other times of the month.

Some experts have seriously questioned the notion that serotonin depletion and carbohydrate cravings motivate binge eating. They cite a number of studies showing that fats and not carbohydrates are the food of choice during most binges. However, when I talk to binge eaters they seem convinced that carbohydrate craving and sugar addiction is real. In fact, some try to control their problem by eliminating sugar completely from their diets, much like an alcoholic going "on the wagon." Although this might seem logical, total deprivation is definitely not the answer. I will show you how to control your cravings and eat sweets in moderation.

HUNGER

Overweight binge eaters have greater and more frequent hunger than overweight nonbinge eaters. This occurs in spite of the fact that overweight individuals in general are less likely to know when they are actually hungry than are people who are not overweight. As I mentioned in the last chapter, your hunger may be more a function of emotions or the availability of food than real hunger.

In spite of this, researchers have measured the gastric capacities of people with binge-eating disorder. Gastric capacity means just what it sounds like—how much your stomach can hold. Chronic overeating results in your stomach being able to hold more. Bulimics have significantly increased gastric capacities. When overweight individuals are tested, binge eaters also have increased gastric capacities but overweight nonbinge eaters do not show this pattern.

When your stomach's capacity is increased, it takes more food to satisfy you. Over time, your binges may increase in size because you rarely feel full with a moderate amount of food.

Ed, a 35-year-old government employee, came to me for help when his weight reached 275 pounds. He had little energy or stamina and suffered from shortness of breath. He had high blood pressure, high cholesterol, and realized that his eating was totally out of control. He reported a history of binge eating that went back several years.

One of Ed's eating problems was that he never felt full. Here is how he described it.

I seem to be hungry most of the time. When I eat a meal, I usually eat very rapidly. I guess that's because I'm so hungry. I usually eat a lot. I've gotten used to very large portions. But,

67

once the meal is over, I really don't feel full. This doesn't make sense since I usually eat about twice as much as I should.

The problem that Ed has with not knowing when he is full is an important one that must be resolved. By eating rapidly, Ed is making the problem worse since it takes about 20 minutes after eating for hunger messages to be turned off by your brain. One of the key concepts in my treatment program is to make you aware of satiety (the feeling of stomach fullness) as well as real physical hunger. Ed learned to slow his eating and began to pay attention to physical sensations of fullness during and after his meal. I am pleased to say that he lost 85 pounds and has con-quered his binge-eating problem.

Now that we have examined why you binge, it's time to do something about it.

CHAPTER 7

....

Getting Ready for a New Life

It is important to begin any program of change with the right mental attitude. Changing patterns of behavior that have been around a long time is a challenge and not a task to be entered into lightly. Change takes commitment and focus. The road to overcoming your binge-eating disorder will be a challenge but not an overwhelming or impossible one. The majority of overweight binge eaters are able to defeat their problem, free themselves from their dependence on food, and lose weight.

....

RESISTANCE TO CHANGE

Even though you may be more than ready to give up your binge eating since it has caused you so much distress, there may be a part of you that resists. Why would this be? Why would any part of your mind want to hold on to a behavior that has kept you from losing weight and that makes you feel so guilty and miserable?

The answer is that your binge eating serves a purpose. Food may be your drug to help you manage depression, anger, tension, and fear. It may represent an enjoyable recreational activity that fills your time and keeps you from being bored with life. It may be an important (or your only) source of personal pleasure and self-gratification. Clients have told me that keeping enough food around the house gives them feelings of comfort and security. Certain foods, such as chocolate, may soothe you like a hot bath or a relaxing massage. No wonder you may unconsciously resent giving up something that provides you so much physical and emotional pleasure and support. Giving up binge eating is like giving up a bad relationship. You crave it so much but you also know how damaging it is for you. In some ways, we want it both ways. We want to continue eating but not experience any of the bad consequences. This is the child in us saying, "I want to grow up and be independent but I don't want to give up the security of my childhood." Unfortunately, this is simply not possible.

HOW IMPORTANT IS FOOD IN YOUR LIFE?

Let's get down to basics. Any resistance you may have is directly related to how important food is in your life. I often ask my clients to list six things that bring them the most emotional or physical pleasure and satisfaction in their lives. I am astounded by the fact that food is frequently in the top three and quite often is number one. These clients are admitting that food is *the* most important element in their lives. This is sad and unfortunate.

This is why, before embarking on this program, you need to take a look at yourself very closely. You need to examine your priorities and values. If we are going to free you from your binge-eating problem, what are we freeing you to do? Overcoming binge eating and losing weight are not the end products of this program. These changes represent the beginning, the beginning of whoever you want to be or have ever wanted to be.

In my experience, clients who succeed the most are those who attribute a special significance to the defeat of their binge-eating disorder. Taking on this challenge represents more than changing one facet of their behavior. Taking control of their eating becomes symbolic of taking control of their lives. They become passionate about change and from this passion comes commitment, motivation, and determination. They strongly believe they can do it and this strong belief makes them try even harder to change, especially when temptation is the greatest.

It is also important to realize that change must be worth the effort. You cannot simply be motivated by the desire to escape from the negative consequences of your problem. Of course, the frustration, guilt, and negative self-esteem that come from binge eat-ing, as well as the disillusionment of repeatedly losing and regaining weight, are reasons enough to want to change. But, change must bring about positive changes as well. There must be significant changes in your day-to-day quality of life or you will not be able to sustain your motivation over the long run.

The promise I make to you is that defeating binge eating is definitely worth it in spite of the fact that you are giving something up. You are letting go of a demon that perhaps has been haunting you for many, many years. The most immediate result that I see in client after client is that they are free, finally free, from their dependence on food. They can now lose weight, keep it off, and get on with their lives.

Douglas, a 26-year-old single copywriter for an ad-vertising agency, successfully conquered his binge-eating disorder while he was still a relatively young man. He had been large since childhood and he had been teased a great deal about his size and weight. His weight and appetite were a continual topic of conversation at home with his parents. It didn't help that a younger brother was slim and could eat any-thing he wanted without gaining an ounce.

Douglas was always self-conscious about his size and developed a very shy, insecure personality. In high school his history teacher took a special interest in him and encouraged Douglas to pursue athletics. The teacher introduced Douglas to the football coach, who saw potential in the young man's large stature. The high school was small and the coach was always on the lookout for students who were either fast or large.

Douglas agreed to try out for the team. Although his size was an asset, Douglas was slow and unsure of himself. Fortunately, his coach was patient and he put Douglas on a vigorous workout program of running, weight training, and dietary restriction. Douglas thrived on his coach's attention. He worked diligently and lost about twenty pounds. He developed strength and endurance and began to feel proud of himself for the first time in his life. During this time, without any extra help, he went from being a C to a B student.

After high school, Douglas went to a small liberal arts college and majored in English. He had a knack for writing and was very creative in his work. He tried out for the college football team but soon found out that college football was highly competitive and lacked the camaraderie of high school sports. He was not enthused about his participation in college football, and after suffering a mild concussion in one of the tryout sessions, he decided that he'd had enough. Without sports, Douglas's weight during college increased dramatically. He gained 38 pounds during his freshman and sophomore years. Although he was studious, Douglas was shy with other people and did not make friends easily. He was a fun-loving, likeable boy, but very reserved around others. He was particularly shy around members of the opposite sex. As he gained weight, his self-esteem and self-confidence plummeted.

Douglas spent a great deal of time alone. He found solace in food and began to binge several times a week. As he gained more weight and his insecurities increased, his binge eating became worse. His eating was out of control. His weight and his binge eating embarrassed and frustrated him, but he was in no mood to do anything about them. He had given up.

After college, Douglas found a job as a copywriter with a regional advertising firm. He had a real talent for fresh ideas and innovative concepts as far as print media ads were concerned. Over the next few years his career flourished even though his personal life was lacking. Although he had two close friends, he spent most of his time alone. He rarely dated and always felt self-conscious about his weight. He continued to feel secretly embarrassed about his binge eating.

His decision to seek help for his binge eating and weight problem was precipitated by two events. His supervisor at work had a heart-to-heart talk with Douglas about his appearance. As Douglas gained more and more weight he became less concerned about his clothing and personal appearance. In addition, he found it extremely difficult to find clothes that fit him. His clothes shopping was limited exclusively to the "big and tall" men shops that catered to the larger sizes. The second impetus for Douglas's coming to see me for help was that he met a young woman with whom he became infatuated. They had never actually dated but worked in the same office and enjoyed long conversations with each other.

Douglas was ready for a change. He felt that he really did not have much of a life. His career had potential but his personal life was going nowhere. He wanted to find a companion in life, get married, and have children. He was a caring, deeply sensitive person who had a lot to offer in a relationship.

After four months of treatment, Douglas gained control of his binge eating and began to lose weight. He was determined to change his life and put every one of my recommendations into practice with enthusiasm. He worked on his self-esteem and body image as well as his eating.

Douglas is a true success case. He overcame his binge eating, which is no longer a problem for him. He lost 78 pounds and began dating Patricia, the woman he met at work. He started working out at a local health club, met new people, and began to come out of his shell. Douglas was able to turn his life around. He developed confidence in himself and no longer felt self-conscious. Even before he began losing weight, he said to me, "Just by getting in control of my eating makes a tremendous difference in how I feel about myself. I didn't think I could do it. You showed me that I could. I feel like I have my life back again. No . . . actually, I feel that my life is just beginning and I can do with it whatever I choose. My life is finally mine to live as I see fit. I can finally start to think about what kind of life I really want. Before I overcame my binge-eating disorder, I was just living life from day to day. I didn't care. I was putting in my time. I guess I thought that's how everybody lives. You taught me to put enthusiasm and passion into my life. You were right. Defeating my binge eating and losing weight were only the first steps. I know now that I will never go back to my old habits. Food will never be that important to me again. I simply won't let it. There is more to my life than being alone and eating. I'm free and I'll never allow myself to be controlled by food again."

I want you to transform yourself just as Douglas did. You *can* have a new life, a new you. Once you take control of your binge eating and begin to manage your weight, you will be free to be the person you were meant to be.

HOW THIS PROGRAM DIFFERS FROM OTHER DIETS YOU'VE BEEN ON

I am sure that what you want out of this program is to overcome your binge-eating problem, lose weight, and be able to keep your weight off and under control. All of these results are possible. However, this is a program of total change and **not a diet.**

You must realize that your major problem, the problem that keeps you from losing weight and keeping it off, is binge eating. Binge eating and not being overweight is the problem we will focus on. Of course, the two are related and as you control your binge eating you will lose weight. You must remember that no diet will help you as long as you binge. This is very important because in the past you have tried to solve your problem through dieting. This program will help you control bingeing and lose weight but changing the binge eating is our first priority.

Because of this, you will not be following a strict diet on this program. This will be new to you at first. Strict diets actually have been your downfall and have been responsible for your binges. There are three forms of dieting that have hurt you in the past. We must change all of these and not allow them to happen ever again. They are:

1. Avoidance of eating for long periods of time
2. Excessive restriction of total number of calories
3. Avoidance of eating "forbidden" foods

To help you avoid these detrimental dieting practices you will be following a very organized food plan in which you will eat six times a day (three meals and three snacks) on a schedule. Although your diet will be a healthy one, it will include a variety of foods. Emphasis will be placed on portion sizes of food rather than calories, although portion control eventually results in a lowering of the calories you are eating each day. I don't want you thinking or worrying about calories or trying to restrict your calories to a low level. You will lose weight once you cease your binge eating and control the portions of the foods you eat.

Finally, there are no lists of "forbidden" foods in this program. Avoidance of certain foods has been one of your problems. It sets up an all-or-nothing phenomenon in which you are either completely avoiding higher-calorie foods or bingeing on them. I will be showing you how to eat your binge foods in moderation. You may not believe this to be possible but, I assure you, it is. In fact, it is not just a possibility, it is a necessary part of your overcoming your binge-eating problem.

WHAT RESULTS YOU CAN EXPECT

If you follow this program with commitment and determination and put all the elements into practice, you will achieve three major changes in your life:

- You will stop binge eating
- You will lose weight
- You will regain control of your life

Studies have shown that the majority of people who follow the guidelines that I am about to share with you show great improvement in their control over food. Most stop binge eating altogether. Some find that, from time to time, under conditions of great stress, they temporarily fall back into their old binge habits. These lapses are both short-term and few and far between.

As you gain control over your binge eating you will begin to lose weight. It is important to remain patient and stay focused on your main problem, binge eating. Successful weight control is a by-product of your success with binge behavior. Do not get caught up with quick weight loss. You will lose weight, but it will be steady and gradual. Remember: fad, rigid, ultra-low-calorie diets are part of your problem. These diets offer false hope, eventual disappointment, and discouragement. They are your enemy.

When you stop binge eating and begin to lose weight you will also notice a drastic change in your life. My program not only shows you how to change your behavior but also how to change your attitude about yourself and your life. You will experience improvements in mood and self-image. You will begin to believe in yourself once again. You'll regain control of your mind and body. You will begin to care about yourself and your life in a much more significant way. You will begin to take care of yourself and make yourself a higher priority. Your life will take on new meaning, purpose, and passion.

Now that you are ready, let's begin your journey to freedom and self-control.

CHAPTER 8

....

Mindful Eating:
The Key to Overcoming
Binge-Eating Disorder

Don't be discouraged by the fact that there are many causes of binge eating. Even though most human behavior is complex, we can still understand and change it. The treatment program I will outline for you is a seven-step plan that attacks binge eating on many fronts. Treatment will focus on your compulsive overeating as well as the thoughts, feelings, and circumstances that trigger it.

In recent years successful treatments for binge eating have been developed and studied in major universities and medical schools around the world. Dr. Christopher Fairburn of Oxford University in England, Dr. Stewart Agras of Stanford University, Dr. G. Terence Wilson of Rutgers University, as well as Dr. Marsha Marcus and Dr. Rena Wing at the University of Pittsburgh School of Medicine have all been at the forefront of developing a successful treatment protocol for binge-eating disorder.

This treatment, known as *Cognitive-Behavioral*

Therapy, has been very effective in helping binge eaters improve markedly. These improvements in binge eating are well maintained over time. Cognitive-Behavioral Therapy focuses on changing negative thought patterns related to self-esteem, all-or-nothing (perfectionistic) attitudes about dieting, and body image. It also concentrates on changing eating behavior by establishing a normalized eating plan and breaking the binge-eating cycle.

The specific goals of Cognitive-Behavioral Therapy in the treatment of binge-eating disorder are to:

- Normalize your eating schedule
- Increase your awareness of what and why you are eating
- Train you to eat "forbidden" foods occasionally and in moderation
- Break your pattern of all-or-nothing, perfectionistic thinking in relation to food
- Improve your self-esteem and body image
- Develop alternative ways to deal with emotional distress

I have been studying the problems of obesity and binge eating for almost 25 years. In that time, I have found that the most efficient way to accomplish the goals of Cognitive-Behavioral Therapy is through a concept known as *Mindful Eating*. Before we begin your treatment program, I will explain how mindful eating can help you change your eating patterns forever.

···

MINDFULNESS: THE KEY TO THE MINDFUL-EATING PROGRAM

The fundamental concept underlying my treatment program is *mindfulness*. Many people are not aware of this term or what it means. If you have heard of it, you probably associate it with meditation and stress management. In fact, Dr. Jon Kabat-Zinn of the University of Massachusetts Medical Center pioneered its well-known use with patients suffering from stress-related medical problems such as hypertension, cancer, and cardiovascular disease.

Mindfulness is not a new idea. It is an ancient concept that is the central component of meditation. Mindfulness is a state of mind that will help you gain control over your emotions, thoughts, and behavior. It will put you back in charge of your eating.

Mindfulness is *awareness*. It is not simply paying attention but a deep, focused awareness of yourself and your surroundings on a moment-to-moment basis. It is paying attention, on purpose.

Most of our eating occurs automatically, without real awareness. This is true whether you are eating low-calorie, nutritious foods or two candy bars. I mentioned earlier that when people binge they often do so in a robotlike, "spaced-out" manner. This state of mind is the exact opposite of mindfulness and one that is designed to keep you feeling out of control. Food is in charge, not you. Together, we can put a stop to this and put you back in control of your eating and your life.

Mindfulness will provide you with the opportunity to change your relationship with food and, eventually, your dependence on food. You will learn to heighten your awareness of every aspect of your life as it relates to food and eating. We will be applying mindfulness to your thoughts and emotions associated with food as well as to your hunger and appetite. To stop binge eating you must first become mindful of your automatic reactions related to food.

THE FOUR ESSENTIAL COMPONENTS OF MINDFULNESS

Mindfulness is a way to listen more closely to your mind and body to increase your understanding of your inner self. It gives you more personal power over your cravings and emotions. It provides a way to observe your mind, to watch your thoughts and feelings without being caught up in them.

Mindfulness is simply a different way of looking at things, a way that will enlighten, strengthen, and empower you. I see it happen to people every day.

The four characteristics of a mindful approach to your eating are:

1. Paying Attention

You must begin to focus your attention on the thoughts, feelings, and circumstances that trigger your desire to eat and make it difficult for you to stop eating. This means paying attention. Paying attention means not allowing yourself to be distracted.

2. Increasing Awareness

Once you begin to pay attention to your eating, you must begin to develop a sense of focused concentration on all aspects of your relationship with food. You must become aware of the details of how, what, where, and why you eat.

3. Focusing on the Present Moment

Mindfulness involves focusing on a particular moment in time. When you eat, you must begin to concentrate exclusively on eating. During a meal, I don't want you to be thinking about what happened earlier in the day or what is going to be happening tomorrow. Neither do I want you to be on automatic pilot, only half aware of what you are doing. This will be a new experience since we live most of our lives in the past and future in a semiconscious state of going through the paces of day-to-day living.

4. Adopting an Observational, Nonjudgmental Attitude

To be mindful is to be an observer, not a judge. With most things in life, we are quick to label and judge. When you are on a diet and you experience hunger (be it physical appetite or emotional craving), you are probably quick to label that experience as "bad." When you judge hunger to be negative you give it power and you begin a struggle that you will surely lose.

I will help you understand that food cravings and hunger are neither good nor bad, they simply exist. They are merely feelings, thoughts, and physical sensations. They are not *you*. They are experiences *within* you. You can choose to react to them and allow them to overwhelm and suffocate you or you can choose to be aware of them and then let them go.

Don't worry if you don't understand all of this now or exactly how it works. Keep an open mind and it will become clear.

THE MINDFUL-EATING PROGRAM

One of the most important ideas behind the Mindful-Eating Program is that you must begin to focus your attention on binge eating, not weight loss. Weight loss is important and is the eventual goal of this program. However, as you know from past experience, your dieting efforts will fail unless you defeat your binge-eating disorder.

This focus on binge eating is very important. In the beginning of the program you must learn to evaluate your progress based on fewer binge-eating episodes as opposed to how much weight you've lost. You must have patience and not try to accomplish too much in a short period of time.

This is a step-by-step program that will attack your binge eating on many fronts. You must go through all of the steps and in the order I present them to you. All the elements of this program are needed for you to be successful.

The Mindful-Eating Program is divided into seven steps:

Step 1   **Mindful-Eating Awareness:** Increasing awareness of hunger and fullness

Step 2   **Mindful Willpower:** Using guided exposure and portion control to overcome binges

Step 3   **Mindful Food Planning:** Establishing a normalized eating pattern

Step 4   **Mindful Emotional Freedom:** Breaking the connection between food and emotions

Step 5   **Mindful Self-Talk:** Changing your perfectionistic and negative thinking

Step 6   **Mindful Body Image and Self-Esteem:** Increasing your feelings of self-worth related to your body and yourself

Step 7   **Mindful Exercise:** Establishing a binge-prevention exercise plan

....

A FINAL WORD ABOUT
YOUR PROBLEM

Before you begin the Mindful-Eating Program I want to say that you are embarking on a program that can change your life. I want you to believe that change is possible. You may be so discouraged by your binge eating that you have lost all hope.

Forget the past. You can regain your confidence. You are not a failure. You just did not know what your problem was all about or what to do about it.

All I am asking of you is total commitment to my seven-step program. I will help you develop a stronger belief in yourself and your ability to succeed. Food does not have to rule your life. You can succeed and you will.

CHAPTER 9

....

Mindful-Eating Awareness

I am now going to teach you how to become more aware of your eating and everything associated with it. This approach may confuse you at first. Most dieters are accustomed to avoiding the thought and sight of food when trying to lose weight. Such avoidance leads to all-or-nothing, perfectionistic thinking, which is at the heart of your binge-eating problem.

You must learn that **food is not your enemy**. Rather, food and eating must become much more important in your life. I don't want you to become obsessed with food, but you must dramatically increase your attentiveness toward what you are eating.

Some of my clients resist this notion. They tell me that they should be able to be "normal" when it comes to eating. They don't want to pay so much attention to what, why, when, where, and how they are eating. Sharon, a 56-year-old schoolteacher, presents a good example of this attitude. Here are her comments:

I have a friend who is as skinny as a rail. When I go to her house, the kitchen is full of cookies, ice cream, and snacks. These foods don't bother her. Her attitude is that she can take them or leave them. She actually has a bag of peanut-butter cookies in her cabinet that's been there for a month. Those cookies wouldn't last in my kitchen for a day! Dr. Miller, if I put all of your advice into practice, when can I be like my friend? When can I be like a person who has never been overweight and who has never had a binge-eating problem?

My answer is that you definitely *can* conquer your binge eating and you *can* lose weight, but you probably will always have to pay more attention to your eating patterns than people who have never had a binge problem. I am not trying to discourage you. *Paying attention* is not the same as obsession. Most of the time, you will not be tempted by your favorite foods and will not be struggling to control your impulses. But awareness and sensitivity to potential binge eating will strengthen you in high-risk situations such as times of severe stress.

You are not being "cured." You are learning to manage and control your binge eating. You may, however, continue to be more sensitive than the average person to food and body weight. This is not necessarily bad if it teaches you to be vigilant about situations that might place you in the path of temptation. Someone who is dealing with an alcohol problem does not necessarily have daily thoughts or fears or temptations about drinking, but, deep down, that person remains aware that the potential for a lapse in self-restraint is there.

....

HOW TO PRACTICE
EATING AWARENESS

There are various ways to increase your awareness of your eating patterns. One of the most typical techniques used in behavior modification programs is known as **self-monitoring**. Self-monitoring consists of keeping a daily written record of what and how much you eat, what time you ate it, where the eating occurred, your thoughts and feelings at the time, and whether or not you considered the eating to be a binge. This is actually a cornerstone of cognitive-behavioral treatment programs for binge eating.

Self-monitoring allows you to analyze your eating pattern in great detail and trains you to become more aware of your eating. In a therapeutic setting, it helps your therapist analyze your binges and evaluate your progress during treatment.

Some people have difficulty being consistent with self-monitoring because it requires a very detailed approach to analyzing behavior. My alternative to self-monitoring is *mindful-eating awareness.*

Mindful-eating awareness is simply applying a

mindful attitude toward eating and the circumstances surrounding it. Remember, as I described in Chapter 8, a mindful attitude is one in which you are:

- Paying attention
- Increasing your awareness
- Focusing on the present moment and the task at hand
- Not allowing yourself to become distracted and lose your focus
- Adopting an observational and nonjudgmental attitude

Mindful-eating awareness means being alert and watchful. You become a curious observer, trying to find out about every aspect of your eating behavior. You are an outside observer looking in.

You may have tried to analyze your binge eating in the past without success. In fact, the process may have been frustrating to you. This is because, as a binge eater, you are too judgmental and critical of yourself and your behavior. You were not just observing but probably were putting yourself down in the process. Also, I am not asking you to observe just your binge eating but all of your eating.

You can develop mindful-eating awareness by practicing the following techniques:

- The Mindful-Eating Style
- The Quiet Meal
- The Raisin Meditation

....

THE MINDFUL-EATING STYLE

The **Mindful-Eating Style** is one in which you pay particular attention each and every time you eat anything, whether it is a meal, a snack, or a binge. Get into the custom of taking a moment or two to adopt a mindful attitude prior to each meal or snack. When you sit down to eat, wait just a moment to contemplate what you are about to do. Calm yourself and relax. Eliminate all other thoughts, concerns, worries, and scheduled activities from your mind. For the next few moments, eating should be the only activity attracting your attention. Keep the past and future out of your mind and focus only on the present moment.

Eating in a mindful way, without distractions, may take some getting used to. We rarely eat mindfully. We hardly ever pay attention to the process of eating. You may be in the habit of sitting in front of your television set while eating, paying very little attention to what is going into your mouth. You and your family may take the opportunity at mealtime to discuss the problems of the day. This habit not only distracts your attention from the meal but also associates eating with tension and frustration. That is certainly the exact opposite of what we are trying to accomplish. When binge eating, you may put your mind on automatic pilot so you are not thinking. That's another way to avoid being mindful.

When you are not mindful, you are not in control.

Remember, mindfulness is the key to being in charge of your eating and it represents the means of access to your new freedom from food.

QUESTIONS TO HELP YOU FOCUS

Let's suppose you are sitting down to a meal. Take a brief time to clear your mind and concentrate on the meal ahead. Relax, and take a deep breath. Slowly exhale. You are not in any hurry. Remind yourself that eating is an important activity in your day and it should not be rushed. Remind yourself that awareness and focus are the keys to your success in overcoming your binge eating.

Look at the food you are about to eat. Take a close look. Silently ask yourself the following questions and think deeply about your answers to each:

What does each item of food look like?
What colors are these foods?
What are the shapes of the foods?
How are the foods arranged on the plate?
How much of each food do I have in front of me?
How big a portion of each food do I have?

As you begin to contemplate these questions, begin eating. I want your eating to be normal so you don't have to take an extraordinarily long time for these mindfulness questions. After you do this a few times, mindful eating will become more automatic and natural. You'll begin to think about the details of the food throughout the meal. Don't think about this as a chore. You are practicing mindful-eating awareness to enhance your enjoyment of the experience and to increase your powers of self-control.

As you begin to eat, pay attention to the food in your mouth. What does the physical presence of that particular food feel like in your mouth? What is the texture of the food? Is it hard? Soft? As you bite into it, what is its taste? What flavors are you experiencing? Think about the experience of chewing each particular food. Focus on the act of swallowing. What is the experience of the food going down your throat and into your body?

In order to pay so much attention to the details of your eating experience, you must eat slowly. This may be a new experience for you. Most people eat very quickly. Studies show that many meals are consumed in as little as five minutes. Take your time and slow yourself down. This is very important.

To convince yourself to eat more slowly you are going to have to convince yourself that eating is an important activity. When you say, "I don't have time to eat slowly," you are saying that other activities in your life are more important than eating. This may have been true in the past, but if you want to overcome binge eating, you must change. I realize that you have certain time constraints as well as responsibilities and obligations. I am not telling you to give all those up. I am simply saying that food and eating must have a higher priority in your life than they had previously.

HUNGER AND SATIETY: AWARENESS OF YOUR INTERNAL SENSATIONS

Although you probably think that part of your problem is an overactive appetite, your difficulty is just the opposite. As a binge eater, you don't know enough about your hunger. You are not as aware of physical hunger as you should be. Part of the reason is that you are confusing physical and emotional hunger. Over the years, your eating has become driven more by external factors (such as stress in your life or the mere presence of food) than internal ones (such as stomach contractions or a feeling of emptiness in your stomach).

In addition to hunger, you must also learn to identify satiety. Satiety is the opposite of hunger; it's a feeling that you are full or satisfied. Studies show that binge eaters cannot usually tell when they are no longer hungry. They do not seem to be able to identify bodily sensations associated with satiety. If these signals are weak or if you are not paying attention to them, you will probably continue to eat until all the food is gone.

You can learn to become more aware of both hunger and satiety. In this chapter I will focus on the physical sensations of hunger and fullness and in a later chapter I'll have more to say about emotional hunger. I am aware that much of your binge eating is triggered by something other than real, physical hunger.

To become more mindful of hunger, take 15 or 20

seconds to think about how you feel before you eat anything. Are you hungry? If so, what does that hunger feel like? Is it a physical sensation? Is your stomach growling? Does it feel "empty"? Are there any special sensations in your throat or mouth? I understand that much of the hunger that triggers binge eating is more emotional than physical. But for now, I want you to develop a better notion of what "real" hunger feels like so you can begin to tell the difference between physical appetite and emotional need.

After you have identified your hunger and how intense it is, begin eating. As you eat, pay attention to changes that occur in your hunger level. At what point are you beginning to feel less hungry? At what point are you no longer hungry? I want you to become an expert on your appetite. To help you judge your level of hunger and satiety, choose one meal a day and rate your hunger (1) before the meal, (2) halfway through, and (3) after you are finished, using the following scale.

The Hunger Awareness Scale

10 ......Starving, need food immediately
9 ......Very, very hungry, unable to think about anything else
8 ......Very hungry, ready to eat now
7 ......Hungry, but could wait a while before eating
6 ......Beginning to feel slightly hungry
5 ......Comfortable (neither hungry nor full)

4 ......Satisfied but not full
3 ......Full with no feelings of hunger
2 ......Very full
1 ......Uncomfortably full, feeling stuffed
0 ......Very uncomfortably full, stomach bloated
and painful

THE QUIET MEAL

An excellent way to practice the Mindful-Eating Style is through the **Quiet Meal**. This is particularly true if you eat most of your meals with other people or if you frequently eat in restaurants. While you can and should eat mindfully at each meal or snack, when others are present, it is difficult and impractical to concentrate your full attention to the look and taste of food as well as to your feelings of hunger and satiety.

This is why you should schedule a Quiet Meal at least once a week (and more often, if you get the opportunity). A Quiet Meal is a meal or snack that you eat in quiet solitude with no distractions from anyone or anything. There should be no one around at the time and you should schedule at least 20 to 30 minutes of uninterrupted time.

This eating occasion could be a full meal or a scheduled snack. Take special effort and attention to prepare this meal. It doesn't have to be elaborate, but you shouldn't just throw something together quickly. During the Quiet Meal you should be sitting down at a kitchen or dining-room table. Take time to prepare the table and surroundings. I want you to be comfortable and relaxed.

When you place the food on the table, make certain that it is arranged in an appealing way on the plate. Whether it is a full meal, a sandwich, or simply a piece of fruit cut up in pieces, I want it to look appetizing. I want you to think that you are worth the effort.

While sitting and looking at the food, think about what you are about to do. Take a deep breath and slowly let it out. Relax. You are going to eat and enjoy your meal but you are going to do it slowly, deliberately, and mindfully.

As you eat, follow the instructions I gave you when discussing the Mindful-Eating Style. Be aware of what the food looks like, what it tastes like, and your experience of hunger and satiety.

One of my most successful clients, Mary, is a 46-year-old woman who schedules a Quiet Meal once every day. Before coming to me for help she had been severely overweight for 20 years. She had tried just about every diet and every weight-control program available. None worked because none of them addressed her real problem: binge-eating disorder. She has been free from binge eating for two years now and is like a totally different person. Once her binge eating was under control she was able to lose 55 pounds and keep them off.

Mary finds the Quiet Meal a soothing, peaceful experience. For her, this mindful-eating time is a symbol of her newly developed power over food. Each day, the Quiet Meal gives her confidence and strengthens her resolve. She usually chooses lunch as her quiet time and takes about 30 full minutes to eat her meal. When she first began doing this, she found herself becoming very impatient. She was not accustomed to eating so slowly and paying so much attention to eating. After a few Quiet Meals, she began to feel more relaxed and actually started to look forward to this experience. Even now, after she has been so successful, the Quiet Meal is an important time for Mary and helps to keep her mindful of everything she eats.

THE RAISIN MEDITATION

The **Raisin Meditation** is a specific technique that will heighten your awareness of food and your reactions to it. I regularly use this with clients to illustrate what mindful-eating awareness is all about.

To begin with, you will need to purchase a small box of raisins for this exercise. Then, find a time when you will be alone and undisturbed for 10 to 15 minutes. With the box of raisins in hand, sit down at your kitchen or dining-room table. Sit in a straight but comfortable position. Place the box of raisins on the table in front of you. Take a deep, full breath and slowly let it out. Clear your mind. For the next few moments, I want you to concentrate on this exercise and nothing else. Take another deep, full breath and slowly let it out.

Try to develop a state of mindfulness by focusing

just on this moment in time. Imagine that the past and future no longer exist, only the present time, and only the next few moments of time. Stay alert and be aware. For the next few moments, you will be an observer of your experiences.

Slowly begin to open the box of raisins. Take out one raisin and then close the box. Hold the raisin in your hand with your palm up and open. Hold it up in front of you so you can see it clearly. Now, look at the raisin. Look at it very closely. I want you to feel a sense of curiosity and wonder about the raisin. Examine its color and its shape. Take your time. Don't hurry. The only thing that matters is this moment in time and what the raisin looks like to you.

Now pick up the raisin and hold it between your thumb and index finger. Take a slow, deep breath and close your eyes. Pay attention to the feeling of the raisin between your fingers. What does it feel like? Gently push against the raisin with your fingers and pay attention to how hard or soft it is. Slowly move the raisin between your fingers and pay attention to its texture and shape. Take your time and do this very slowly. Don't be in a hurry.

Next, gradually bring up your hand to position the raisin just under your nose. Deeply inhale and smell the raisin. Take in its aroma. Take your time and savor it. Be aware of it.

Now, move your hand down to your mouth and, very gently, place the raisin in your mouth and let it go. Do not chew or swallow it—just place it in your mouth and leave it there. Pay attention to the physical sensation of having the raisin in your mouth. Think about it. After that, begin to move the raisin around in your mouth. Be aware of the contact it makes with your tongue, your gums, the roof of your mouth, the inside of your cheeks, and your teeth. Take your time and pay attention to the experience.

As you are doing this, pay attention to any other thoughts and feelings you are experiencing. Just be aware of them. Don't get caught up with them. Your prime focus should be on the raisin. However, if you are thinking, "This seems silly. I wonder how this is going to help me stop binge eating?" be aware of the thought, acknowledge it, and then let it go. Refocus your mind on the raisin in your mouth.

Next, maneuver the raisin around in your mouth so that it is located between your teeth, as if you are about to bite into it. Hold it there, paying attention to the contact between your teeth and the raisin. Gently move it from side to side between your teeth.

Now it's time to take a bite. Very slowly and deliberately, I want you to bite down on the raisin. As you bite into it, pay attention to the feel of the raisin against your teeth. Be aware of taste sensations that you are experiencing. What is the flavor? Think about what is happening. Before you bite into it again, make certain that you have been aware of the total experience of the raisin.

Continue to chew the raisin, but do so slowly, deliberately, and with awareness. Be very conscious of what you are doing and what you are experiencing.

Do not allow anything else to distract you. Focus and concentrate.

At some point in the chewing process, you will be ready to swallow the raisin. I want you to be aware of the exact second that you decide to swallow it. Since such actions are automatic most of the time, it will be necessary for you to pay a great deal of attention to what is happening in your mouth.

When you begin to swallow the raisin, think about what it feels like as it goes down your throat. Keep concentrating on it as long as the experience lasts. When the raisin is gone, focus on your thoughts and feelings. What is in your mind? What are you saying to yourself about the Raisin Meditation? What are you thinking or feeling about what you have just experienced?

If you're like many of my clients, you might be thinking something like, "I don't think I've ever really tasted a raisin until now. I didn't realize there was so much to it." Many people also report, "I've had entire meals that I didn't get as much satisfaction out of as that raisin." In fact, studies show that you can eat a meal in as little as five or 10 minutes with very little enjoyment. During this mindfulness session, you are spending about the same amount of time eating one little raisin!

One woman said to me, "If I ate everything like that, I'd never overeat." This is just the point. She hit the nail on the head. Mindful eating is a key to your success and this exercise makes the point very clearly. That is not to say that you must eat everything this slowly and deliberately, but it does show how mindful eating gives you a totally different experience than your normal eating pattern.

Remember, mindful, slow, deliberate eating is the opposite extreme of binge eating. During binge eating, you are eating very rapidly and paying very little attention to what you are doing. Your impulses are driving you and you are out of control. Mindful eating as demonstrated by the Raisin Meditation will help you develop more control over food to put an end to your binge eating.

ONE FINAL BIT OF ADVICE

Remember how your mother told you to eat everything on your plate to keep children from starving around the world? Well, to increase eating mindfulness and practice your determination every day, I want you to leave one morsel of food on your plate. At one meal a day, get into the habit of leaving one mouthful of food on your plate. Make sure it is the food you are enjoying the most at that particular meal. This is a very simple act, but it shows that you are aware of what you are doing. It also proves to you on a daily basis that you are in control of food and that it does not control you.

CHAPTER 10

·······························

Mindful Willpower

Y<small>ou</small> can also apply the concept of mindfulness to develop greater willpower over food. When you think of willpower, what comes to your mind? Self-discipline? Self-control? Reason over emotion? Doing the right thing? Inner strength? Determination?

Think of willpower as the power of choice. It is not "doing the right thing" all the time but having the ability to freely choose. It is the opposite of the out-of-control feeling you have prior to and during a binge.

I often present the following hypothetical situation to those who seek my help.

Let's suppose that I had special magical powers. Because of these powers, I could promise you absolute and total willpower. You would always do the right thing. You would always do everything that is good and healthy for you. Would you want this gift? Would you accept it?

Interestingly enough, about two-thirds of those I ask say, "No." The reason they give is that they would not feel human. Part of our human nature that most of us are not willing to give up is our freedom of choice. We do not want to be robots. However, since we are less than perfect, the price we pay for freedom of choice is fallibility. We make the wrong choices from time to time as part of our nature.

I want you to think of willpower as self-management. Managing your impulses toward food is a skill you can learn. Everyone can learn to have more self-restraint and to avoid being out of control. One of the best ways to learn self-management and apply it to your eating is through the concept of mindfulness.

Self-management is a positive quality that is developed more by paying attention to the times you overcome food cravings than by focusing on your binge episodes. Let me tell you a story to illustrate this point.

THE MINDFUL GOLF LESSON

Living on Hilton Head Island, a resort and retirement community just off the coast of the low country of South Carolina, gives me an occasional opportunity to play golf. I am an average golfer with the usual ups and downs in my game. Several years ago I sought the help of a local golf professional to improve my game. He was an older, seasoned veteran of the game with a reputation for being a wise and insightful teacher.

My major problem for which I was seeking his assistance was a slice. If you don't play golf, a slice means that when you hit the ball it curves to the right (usually landing in the woods or a body of water) instead of going straight. Needless to say, this is an extremely frustrating state of affairs to say nothing of what it does to your score.

I met my golfing guru on the practice range one bright and sunny morning. He instructed me to hit a few balls so he could observe my swing. I proceeded to hit six balls in a row, all of which curved to the right and landed amid several large live oak trees. I then stopped and waited for my instructor to tell me what I was doing wrong. He said nothing but, instead, motioned me to continue hitting golf balls.

I did as I was instructed and hit several more balls into the woods. Still, he said nothing. I was becoming frustrated and impatient and began mentally questioning my choice of golf teacher.

Finally, I hit a ball that went perfectly straight. It was a glorious shot that soared high and far. It was only then that he exclaimed, "STOP! Your lesson will now begin." I didn't know what to think until he asked me a profound question for which I had absolutely no answer. He looked directly at me and asked, "What did you just do to hit that ball straight?" After a moment of thought I realized that I had no earthly idea. He continued, "If you don't know what it takes to hit a straight shot, you will never improve. Learning to avoid a slice tells you very little. Your lesson will focus on what you are doing, thinking, and feeling when you hit a good shot."

Although my good shots were few and far between, he instructed me to pay particular attention to what was happening whenever I hit the ball straight. He wanted me to pay attention and be aware. He wanted me to pay attention to the moment of the swing and what was taking place. In essence, he wanted me to be mindful. He wanted me to practice and play mindful golf.

Most golfers are acutely aware of how far or how straight the ball goes but could tell you very little about the process of making the shot. Successful golf professionals who play on tour could tell you a great deal about what is happening each time they hit the ball. That's exactly why they are so successful.

LEARNING THE SECRETS OF YOUR SUCCESS

After my golf lesson, it dawned on me that the philosophy behind my instructor's teachings applied equally as well to willpower over food. Colleen, a 38-year-old paralegal and mother of two, consulted me about a long-standing binge-eating problem. She had always been overweight by about 20 pounds but, over the past two years, had taken on a new job and added 30 more pounds to her weight. She binged about four to five days a week, eating mostly sweets.

When I first began helping her, she described her binges in great detail, telling me what she ate, how much she ate, and how guilty and remorseful she felt afterward. After hearing about three or four of these episodes, I asked her to tell me about any occurrences during which she was tempted to eat but resisted.

At first, she insisted that such experiences never happened. With further prodding from me, she finally admitted that occasionally she wants to eat but is able to resist. I asked her to give me an example. Colleen remembered that about three weeks ago she bought a large bag of M&M candies while shopping. She arrived home, unpacked her groceries, and opened the bag of candy. She had been trying to diet and knew she shouldn't be eating. She felt that she couldn't help herself. She poured several M&Ms into her hand and ate them quickly. As she began to eat more, she hesitated. Apparently, a battle was going on in her head. For some reason she decided not to continue eating and emptied the bag into her garbage disposal.

After her description of this incident, I asked Colleen the same type of question that my golf instructor had posed to me, "Colleen, what did you do to resist eating more candy?" She had no clue. She had not been paying attention to her success. She had not even considered it a significant event. In fact, she was surprised by my question because she thought I would want to ask her why she ate the one handful of candy. In her mind, this incident was an example of her lack of willpower.

This notion of examining successful self-restraint and redefining partial self-restraint as success may be foreign to you. You may never have considered it. You may never have given yourself credit for it. Your thinking has been negative about your eating experiences, whether good or bad.

In addition, your definition of success is also faulty. You may always have defined success as weight loss. You must change all that and begin to focus on your behavior. Remember, binge eating is the problem that is keeping you from losing weight. You will lose weight but only when you begin to overcome your binge-eating disorder. You'll know when you're getting better when you begin to resist your favorite high-calorie foods.

HOW TO PRACTICE MINDFUL WILLPOWER

In order to strengthen your powers of self-restraint you must be mindful of your successes and partial successes. You must pay attention and be aware of the times when you (1) resist tempting food altogether or (2) partially resist tempting food by eating only some of it. If you typically stop eating when all of the tempting food is gone, then, in the beginning, you should analyze those times when there is even a small amount of food left.

Because of your perfectionistic, all-or-nothing thinking it may be difficult for you to view partial self-restraint as a "success" experience. To you, one M&M is as bad as a whole bag. You must learn to challenge this idea. For now, just follow my guidelines and do the best you can. I'll have more to say about this in Chapter 14.

Let's be a little more specific about mindful willpower. Whenever you refrain from eating fully or partially in a situation that would normally be a binge for you, I want you to go through the following routine:

1. Quickly stop whatever you are doing
2. Find a place where you can be alone for a few moments
3. Close your eyes and enter into a state of mindfulness
4. Focus on the moment and block out all other thoughts
5. Pay attention and be aware
6. Closely observe what you were thinking, feeling, and doing at the time you overcame your craving
7. Closely observe what you are thinking and feeling now that you have been successful

....

WHAT SHOULD YOU
BE LOOKING FOR?

Clients often say to me, "Exactly what am I supposed to be looking for?" Since they rarely stop to think about "success" experiences, they have no experience in analyzing these opportune moments.

This is exactly the question I had when my golf instructor asked me what I had done in order to hit the golf ball straight. Even when I thought about it, I didn't know what to look for. Even when I tried to relive the moment in my imagination, I still had difficulty. I finally began to understand when my instructor told me what other golfers had noticed when they hit their best shots.

Even though everyone's source of willpower is different, it will help you at first if I share the success experiences of others with you. Let me begin by telling you about a very interesting series of studies conducted in the 1980s by Dr. Walter Mischel, a psychologist specializing in self-control.

....

THE MARSHMALLOW STUDY

Dr. Mischel was interested in studying how young children naturalistically, without any special training, resist temptation. He devised an experiment in which children were individually placed in a room with a plate of marshmallows. Each child was then instructed to try to resist eating the marshmallows for as long as they could.

Afterward, the children were interviewed to see what they were thinking about during the experiment. He found that the children who successfully resisted eating the marshmallows were thinking "cool" thoughts such as, "These marshmallows are puffy like clouds." They were consciously redirecting the focus of their attention away from the taste of the food.

The children who did not resist and ended up eating the marshmallows were thinking "hot" thoughts such as, "These marshmallows look yummy and chewy." They failed to distract their attention and inadvertently heightened their cravings by focusing on the anticipation of what the food would taste like.

In fact, the children who resisted seemed to be consciously fighting "hot" thoughts with "cool" ones. The children who did not resist were not fighting at all. They simply were being carried away by their "hot" thoughts.

This study emphasizes that willpower is an active, skillful process. Willpower involves actively engaging in specific thought patterns that move your mind away from food. It is not simply a matter of "toughing it out." These thought patterns can be learned and practiced so that during a temptation you can go through a preplanned mental willpower drill that will help you overcome your food craving.

....

WHAT MY CLIENTS HAVE TAUGHT ME ABOUT WILLPOWER

I have asked hundreds of women and men with binge-eating problems to examine their success experiences in this manner. I believe that what they have learned about their inner strengths may be of help to you. By sharing with you what they discovered about themselves, I will be setting you on a path of your own self-discovery—a discovery of the secrets of your own strength, determination, and willpower. The amazing fact is that it's been there all the time waiting for you to find it. You've just never looked before:

I can divide the willpower thoughts and images of my clients into eight separate categories. They are as follows:

1. Thoughts reminding you of past success (for example, either mentally reliving a time when you were tempted to eat but didn't or thinking about all of the time and effort you have put into your exercise program)
2. Thoughts related to a strong belief in yourself (for example, practicing a prescripted pep talk such as, "I am a strong person and I know I can do this")
3. Thoughts related to specific motivators for weight loss and appetite control (for example, high blood

pressure, diabetes, lack of energy and stamina, or the desire to regain control of your life)

4. Distracting thoughts or actions (for example, imagining that the fat in the cheese is poison to your system or getting out of the house for a while)

5. Thoughts related to emotional control (for example, turning negative emotions into positive energy by insuring that you become more determined in the face of adversity)

6. Thoughts related to alternative actions (for example, any activity that might fill the need that you are experiencing such as taking a hot bath in order to feel calm and soothed)

7. Thoughts related to your personal pride and self-worth (for example, "I am better than this")

8. Thoughts related to a successful future (for example, visualizing yourself three months from now, at a lower weight, feeling strong, confident, and full of energy)

THE WILLPOWER JOURNAL

Once you discover what you were thinking and feeling during your success experience, it is important to write it down. I suggest you purchase a small notebook or journal for this purpose. This will be your Willpower Journal. Each time you overcome temptation (either fully or partially), you should get out your journal and record your answers to the following questions:

- Exactly what were you saying to yourself? What words, phrases, or sentences were going through your mind?
- How would you describe your feelings at the time?
- What visual images were affecting you?
- What specifically did you do?

Let me give you an example from Patricia's journal. Patricia is a 24-year-old graduate student, majoring in business management. Her goal was to work for a large corporation for a few years and then start her own business. Although she was a bright and conscientious student she found the demands of graduate school very difficult.

When stressed or under time demands for important school projects, she found solace in food. Eating became a diversion that kept her from dealing with her anxiety and self-doubt about her competence. She wanted to do well in school and eventually succeed in her career goals, but an inner voice kept telling her that she wasn't good enough or smart enough. She kept having to fight the feeling that she just didn't have what it takes to make it.

She had always had a bit of a weight problem but now her binge eating was adding up. In her first year of graduate school she gained 18 pounds. She was binge eating at least two to three times a week, mostly at night alone when she felt stressed out, lonely, or inadequate. Food soothed and tranquilized her. She would often get into bed with her favorite brand of chocolate ice cream, pull the covers around her, and feel safe, secure, and soothed. At least temporarily. After she had finished the quart container of ice cream she invariably felt terrible. Guilt, remorse, self-hatred, and depression followed.

When she consulted me, she had recently gained 10 more pounds, was barely maintaining an acceptable average at school, and was suffering from depression and panic attacks. She was desperate.

Patricia was so negative about herself and her life that she totally rejected my positive willpower approach when I first discussed it with her. I had to proceed slowly. With patience, along with her desperate desire to change, Patricia finally agreed to try my approach. Little by little, she discovered that she did, indeed, possess inner strength and determination. She did have willpower after all.

She agreed to purchase a small notebook to serve as her Willpower Journal. She started slowly, having difficulty figuring out what was going through her head when she did resist temptation. With practice, she began to look forward to writing in her journal. Her journal entries finally persuaded her that she did, indeed, have willpower. She discovered the secret of her success and gradually began to believe in herself once again. Believe me, it was a joy to see.

There is nothing magical about this process. It simply takes time and patience. Just as Patricia learned, you must believe that:

YOU DEFINITELY HAVE WILLPOWER!
YOU JUST HAVE TO
KNOW WHERE TO LOOK FOR IT.

After four months of help, Patricia became a different person. Her binge eating diminished until she finally was able to give it up completely. She felt stronger and more confident in herself and her future. She lost 29 pounds and had more energy and confidence than she had ever felt.

She was so excited about her new outlook that she wanted me to share some of the entries in her Willpower Journal to help others attain the success and personal freedom that she was experiencing. She is quite an inspiration. When I contacted her four years afterward, she had maintained her weight loss and had only binged three times within four years. These episodes occurred at times of unusual family stress and she was able to get back in control of her eating each time. She had graduated with a master's degree in business administration, was working as an assistant manager in a large textile firm in North Carolina, and was expecting a promotion within the next few weeks.

Here is an entry from Patricia's journal. Notice that she divided her journal into the "Words," "Feelings," "Images," and "Actions" that occurred whenever she successfully overcame food cravings and prevented a binge.

Episode 1

Tuesday evening, 10:00 P.M., feeling restless, bored, tense. Supposed to be studying for Economics test on Friday but can't keep my mind on it. Feeling negative and thinking, "I'm no good at this. I hate economics. I'll probably get the lowest grade in the class." Decided to telephone for a pizza delivery even though I had just eaten a very satisfying dinner at 7:30. Picked up the phone to order a large sausage pizza, dialed the number, then hung up and decided not to do it.

Willpower Analysis:

Words "You've done so well for the last two weeks, you can't blow it now. I'm better than this. I can control myself. I am not going to let food control me anymore. I want to be free from all of this. I want FREEDOM." (At this point, the word "freedom" kept coming into my mind. I saw it in big, red, neon letters.)

Feelings Anger at myself for letting this happen. Anger at allowing my thoughts about the test become so negative. I was trying to turn my anger into strong determination.

Images A clear image of myself in the future, having successfully finished my degree. I am looking trim and fit and in control.

Actions I called Janet, my closest friend, to talk about what just happened. She was very supportive (as I knew she would be) and helped me to stay in a strong, positive state of mind.

....

YOUR WILLPOWER DRILL

After keeping your Willpower Journal for a while, you will begin to see patterns developing. You will begin to discover the specific secrets of your willpower. It is at this point that you can begin to develop Willpower Drills—specific mental rituals that can strengthen you in times of temptation. Rather than wait for positive thoughts and images to come into your mind when you need them, I am suggesting that you routinely rehearse them for use in times of trouble.

Your Willpower Drill can take the form of a word, a phrase, a sentence, an idea, a visual image, a symbol, or an action. It should be prearranged and rehearsed often so you can automatically bring it to mind when you need it. It's just like having a familiar prayer that you say to yourself to strengthen your resolve. You may be familiar with the serenity prayer used by members of Alcoholics Anonymous. Members know this short but meaningful prayer by heart and recite it whenever they are tempted to drink. It goes like this:

The Serenity Prayer

God, grant me
The serenity to accept the things I cannot change,
Courage to change the things I can, and
Wisdom to know the difference.

119

Choose your own Willpower Drill based on your Willpower Journal entries or on what you know will help strengthen you. Here are some examples from clients of mine.

Words:

Power
Strength
Freedom

Sentences:

I am stronger than the craving.
I am in control, not the food.
I know I can do this.
Self-restraint is symbolic of regaining control of my life.

Images:

A picture of yourself at a lower weight.
An image of yourself projected 30 minutes ahead in time, having successfully overcome the temptation.
An image of yourself involved in some form of physical activity, feeling fit, trim, and energetic.

Symbols:

Visualizing the color red for strength
Visualizing the color blue for peace and serenity
Imagining a sunrise as representing a new day and
a new you

Once you have written out your Willpower Drill, practice it every day. These words or images will become symbolic of your inner strength and determination. Consciously bring them to mind whenever you are tempted to binge. Continue to keep your Willpower Journal and to update your Willpower Drill from time to time.

CHAPTER 11

The Mindful Eater's Food Plan

One of the most important goals of your new food plan is to establish a normalized eating schedule. Erratic, haphazard eating makes binge eating more likely because it disrupts the normal physiological controls of eating. Regularly scheduled meals teach your body to know when it is really hungry and will put you more in touch with your feelings of fullness once eating has begun. Eating on a schedule also begins to break the connection between food and emotions.

While you will be eating on a schedule, this is not a rigid diet. Overly restrictive dieting will make your binge problem much worse than it already is. This is a very important point that you must consider carefully. Because of your all-or-nothing thinking, you have a history of going on diets that emphasize very low calories, forbidden foods, and strict dietary rules. You may have taken liquid formulas or diet pills. Such approaches will never work for you for three reasons. First, they strengthen your perfectionistic thoughts. Second, they lead you to believe that you are not strong enough to overcome your binge eating and weight problems on your own. Third, they encourage you to avoid the foods you enjoy and not learn to deal with them.

To normalize your eating, you must organize and structure *how often* you eat, *when* you eat, and *where* you eat. Most diets you have been on in the past probably focused exclusively on *what* you eat. While the quality and quantity of your food is important as far as your binge eating is concerned, it is less important than the circumstances surrounding your eating and your reasons for eating.

All of the experts who treat binge-eating problems agree that:

**A SCHEDULED EATING PLAN IS
THE MOST IMPORTANT WAY TO
COMBAT BINGE EATING.**

HOW OFTEN YOU SHOULD EAT

As a chronic dieter you probably have a tendency to skip meals. This is a big mistake because it sets you up for hunger. The typical binge eater/dieter eats very little in the morning, often skipping breakfast. You may not have much of an appetite in the morning. Lunch may be light in order to save on calories. By late afternoon, you are probably quite hungry since you have had so little to eat during the day.

By 4:30 in the afternoon, if you're having a hectic or stressful day, you are a prime candidate for binge eating. If you work, your high-risk time may be when you first come home after your workday. You probably make a beeline to the refrigerator and because you are hungry, tired, and stressed out, your dieting resolve goes out the window.

The acronym HALT is often used in 12-step programs such as Alcoholics Anonymous or Overeaters Anonymous. The letters refer to Hungry, Angry, Lonely, and Tired. When these feelings occur, you are supposed to stop and consider that you are in a high-risk situation. Any of these feelings alone or in combination can trigger binge eating. One certain way to change this pattern is to set up an eating plan that is designed to help you avoid hunger. The best way to do that is to eat several times a day.

I want you to eat six times each and every day without fail. You should eat three meals—breakfast, lunch, and dinner—and three between-meal snacks a day. You may resist this pattern at first since you are accustomed to skipping meals. If you consider food and eating as your problem, as the enemy, then you will want to avoid it. Just remember that by avoiding meals, you are actually making a binge more likely.

If you worry that all of this eating will cause you to gain weight, I can assure you that it will not. First of all, although you will be eating more frequently, you will be eating smaller portions. Second, eating more frequently actually helps you burn more calories through a process known as dietary thermogenesis. Every time you eat, your body works harder to digest the food and break down the nutrients. This causes your metabolism to rise by 15 to 25 percent for one to three hours after you eat. Dietary thermogenesis occurs even if you eat as little as a 100-calorie snack. By eating more frequently you are not only controlling your binge eating but you are burning many more calories as well.

WHEN YOU SHOULD EAT

Your meals and snacks should be spaced throughout the day so that you are never going more than three to four hours without eating. You should schedule your eating at specific times and stick to those times unless something very unusual disrupts your schedule. A typical meal schedule would look something like this:

7:30 A.M.	Breakfast
10:30 A.M.	Mid-morning snack
12:45 P.M.	Lunch
3:30 P.M.	Afternoon snack
6:30 P.M.	Dinner
10:00 P.M.	Late-night snack

Of course, your exact eating times may differ from this schedule because of your family and work schedule. It is perfectly okay to have a different eating schedule each day or on the weekends as long as you include six eating times and *as long as it is planned at least a day in advance*. A very important point for you to remember is that once your schedule is set you must follow it to the letter.

Meal and snack times *must* take precedence over any other activity in the day. This is extremely important if you are to succeed. I realize that occasionally an activity may occur, such as an unplanned business meeting with your boss or an emergency situation, that will interfere with your schedule. When this happens, make the best of it, but as soon as possible (hopefully, by the next meal or snack), you should be right back on your schedule.

You must realize that until you become accustomed to eating this way you might allow other commitments and activities to interfere. This is especially true if you are a person who is always doing for others and always ready to say "yes" even though you are inconvenienced. You must start looking out for yourself and your own needs. For this system to work for you, you must make eating regular meals a priority. Actually, I should say, a necessity.

At first, many binge eaters resist an eating schedule. I'll never forget a client of mine named Elizabeth who wanted no part of a scheduled meal plan. Elizabeth was in her mid-50s, the mother of two grown children, the grandmother of two, and someone who was very active in community groups and organizations. She also helped her husband part-time, doing accounting work at his commercial contracting business. When I first mentioned the importance of a regular eating schedule, Elizabeth's reaction was, "There is absolutely no way I could eat on a schedule. Dr. Miller, you don't realize what my life is like. I have meetings all the time and I'm just too busy to eat with any regularity."

Just as she had finished telling me this, her wristwatch alarm went off. She apologized for the distraction and explained that she sets her watch to go off four times a day because she has to take medication on a schedule. My reply was, "On a schedule?" "Why, yes," she said, "taking my medication just as my doctor prescribed it, on a regular schedule, is very important to me." Interestingly enough, until I pointed it out to her, Elizabeth saw no discrepancy between her unwillingness to eat meals on a schedule and her determination to take her medicine on a schedule. The difference was a matter of priority.

After more discussion, I convinced Elizabeth that eating meals and snacks at regular intervals was just as important to her binge-eating problem as taking her medicine was to her blood pressure. In fact, she found it helpful to view her binge-eating disorder as a disease that needed precise, organized treatment just like any other medical condition. She realized that if she kept other activities from interfering with her taking medicine, she could do the same thing with meals.

Remember that setting up a meal/snack schedule will not do any good unless normalized eating becomes a major priority in your life. When you allow other activities to interfere, you are saying that solving your binge-eating problem is not important, that it doesn't matter. Overcoming binge eating takes commitment, effort, and action. It does not require a superhuman effort, but it does demand changes in your life. Change is difficult but the rewards of such change will be great. You'll be free from your dependence on food and, once and for all, be able to lose weight and keep it off.

WHERE YOU SHOULD EAT

Where you should eat and what is going on while you are eating is also an important element of controlling your eating. Your goal is to make eating meals and snacks a "pure" experience. By this I mean that eating should be a distinct activity in your day that is separated from other activities. It must be a mindful event that you are paying attention to.

In order to accomplish this, you must eat in places designed for eating such as your kitchen table, dining-room table, or at a table in a restaurant. This is the only way you can really pay attention to what you are doing. This is the only way you can practice the Mindful-Eating Awareness that I discussed in Chapter 9. So, most of the time, you should avoid eating in other locations such as on the sofa, in your favorite lounge chair, in the car, in your bed, or standing up (at the kitchen counter or in front of the refrigerator). You don't have to be perfect with this plan so don't worry if, because of a hectic schedule, one day you are eating a banana as a snack in your car on the way to meet someone.

You must also begin to separate other distracting activities from your eating behavior. It is not possible to be mindful about your eating if you are also watching television, doing paperwork, or reading. **Eating is an important activity** and it should not be secondary to something else. It deserves its own time and space.

The other reason to give eating a separate and distinct place in your life has to do with *conditioned hunger*. When you eat in front of the television set, television viewing becomes associated with eating. After many, many associations, watching television becomes a trigger for your appetite. This is called conditioned hunger and it can be as strong as real hunger. If you eat in many situations while involved in many other activities, you have developed conditioned hunger to many things.

This is very much like a smoker who is trying to quit. Smoking has been conditioned to many other activities such as drinking coffee or having an alcoholic drink. A cup of coffee will automatically trigger cravings for a smoke.

The only way you can break the cycle of conditioned hunger is to separate all other activities from meal and snack times. This sounds simple but it may represent a major change in your life. You may find yourself resisting this change. You may think, "I understand what you're saying but this just wouldn't work for me. I'm too set in my ways. Besides, I can make this program work without doing this." You must understand that eating on a schedule, in a particular place, under quiet, calm circumstances is a major key to this program. The more exceptions you make, the less likely this program will work for you.

Change is difficult but you can do it. Just give it a chance. After the first few days, the changes will become natural to you. I've seen it happen time and time again. And, because of these changes, I've seen hundreds of people free themselves from the chains of food dependence. Binge eating has become a thing of the past.

Even my most successful clients experience resistance to change at first. Some of this resistance is due to fear. Giving up anything that you are dependent on is frustrating. Even though food is your problem, binge eating serves a purpose. You hate yourself for doing it but it is an integral part of your life. It's like a bad personal relationship in which you know someone that you love is damaging to you but you cannot seem to resist the pull of their attraction.

Once you make eating a "pure" experience, fewer and fewer activities trigger your thoughts about food. You'll be able to watch television, for example, without feeling a desire to eat. You'll arrive home from work and not think about food. Your goal is to train your mind and body to anticipate eating only at specific times of day and in specific rooms of the house.

Marcia, a 63-year-old widow, came to me a few years back for help with her weight. She had gained about 30 pounds since her husband died two years previously. She had tried a number of diets and weight-loss programs but nothing seemed to work. After a careful analysis of her condition I discovered that she had all of the characteristics of binge-eating disorder and that this problem was preventing her from losing weight. I started her on my program. When we discussed restricting her eating to the kitchen or dining-room table, she resisted.

Living alone, she was in the habit of eating her meals on a tray in front of the television set. Since her husband's death the television had become her companion. She often watched favorite programs during meals and, as a result, paid little attention to what or how much she was eating. She complained that if she had to eat by herself at the table, doing nothing but eating, she would feel bored and lonely.

I certainly understood Marcia's reaction. I had heard this complaint before. However, I convinced her that this method of eating was an essential key to breaking her binge-eating habit. Eating should not be a boring chore. I want you to enjoy the act of eating. In Marcia's case I encouraged her to make a special effort to set the table in an attractive manner, perhaps making sure there are flowers on the table. I also encouraged her to dine with others more often by inviting friends to lunch or dinner or eating out with them in restaurants. When eating alone, pleasant, relaxing music helps. I suggested that she listen to the radio or buy some special audiotapes or CDs.

It is certainly okay to have a pleasant conversation with someone or to enjoy relaxing music while you are eating. You want to avoid activities that are so disrupting or that take so much of your attention that you are not able to be mindful of how you are eating and what you are eating.

Also, make certain that mealtime is a pleasant, relaxing time. Unfortunately, many families use the dinner hour to discuss all of the problems of the day. This is a very bad idea. It associates eating and food with stress and anxiety. That's just what we want to avoid. Such problems should be discussed before or after the meal with mealtime being considered a "time out" from the day's worries. Think of all six eating times each day as a time to refocus and relax.

In fact, that's where Mindful-Eating Awareness comes into play. Mindfulness is concentrating on the present moment and letting go of the past and future at least for that moment. You should look forward to meal and snack times not only for the nutrition for your body but also for the renewal of your mind and spirit.

WHAT YOU SHOULD EAT

Before I discuss what you should eat, let me remind you again that the Mindful-Eating Program is *not* a diet. Its goal is to help you overcome binge eating.

Once that occurs, you will be able to focus your full attention on weight loss without binge eating being an obstacle.

You should concentrate most of your attention on eating regularly scheduled meals slowly and without distractions. You must avoid rigid diets. You must feel that food choices are yours to make. I don't want you counting calories or fat grams or following restrictive menu plans. In fact, as you will discover in the next chapter, I even want you to eat your binge foods from time to time. Don't panic. I will show you how to do this in a controlled way so that you are eating these foods only occasionally and only in moderation. This is what a normal eating pattern is all about.

I don't want you thinking in terms of eating a certain number of calories each day. I will show you how to reduce calories moderately without worrying about calories. I know this is a new way of doing things for you, but you must trust me. Low-calorie dieting has not worked for you in the past and it will not work for you now. It is part of the problem, not the solution.

You will be controlling your overall food intake in two ways. First, you will be eating at regularly scheduled times and only at those times. Second, you will be controlling serving sizes. Portion control is one of the prime ways to control what you eat without becoming obsessive about calorie restriction.

....

PORTION CONTROL

Portion management requires measuring cups, measuring spoons, and a good food scale. As you measure and weigh foods each day you will learn what ½ cup of cooked rice, ¾ cup of cereal, or 3 ounces of chicken looks like. After a while, you'll become a good judge of portion sizes. Using mental imagery to picture what specific serving sizes look like is extremely helpful. For example,

- 3 ounces of cooked meat, chicken, or fish is about the size of a deck of cards
- 8 ounces of cooked meat is about the size of a small paperback book
- 5 ounces of cooked meat, chicken, or fish is equal to 1 cup
- 1 cup of cereal, chopped vegetables, or diced fruit is the size of your clenched fist
- ½ cup of cooked pasta or rice fits into an ice cream scoop
- 1 ounce of cheese is about the size of four dice
- 1 teaspoon of margarine or mayonnaise is about the size of the top joint of your thumb
- 1 ounce of nuts, small candy, or raisins fits easily into the palm of your hand
- 1 ounce of pretzels or chips fits into two open cupped hands

The following is a list of everyday foods and the portion sizes that I would recommend. In many cases I provide a range of sizes to accommodate individual appetite and choice. The ranges are also designed to keep you from becoming too rigid in your thinking about food.

Bread	1 slice or 1 roll
Cereal	½ to 1 cup
Rice	½ to ¾ cup
Pasta	¾ to 1 cup (cooked)
Potato	½ to 1 medium sized
Vegetables (raw, leafy)	1 to 1½ cup
Vegetables (cooked, chopped)	½ to 1 cup
Vegetable juice	6 to 8 ounces
Fruit (whole)	1 piece
Fruit (chopped)	½ to ¾ cup
Fruit juice	6 to 8 ounces
Milk (1% or skim)	8 ounces
Yogurt	1 cup
Cheese (hard)	1 to 1½ ounces
Cottage cheese	½ cup
Lean meat	3 to 5 ounces
Fish	4 to 6 ounces
Poultry	3 to 5 ounces

Serving sizes for snack foods, ice cream, and foods that are higher in calories and fat are included in the next chapter on binge foods. For foods that are not included here, check the product label for the amount considered to be a standard serving size. Nowadays, all products carry this information along with calories and fat grams.

....

GENERAL NUTRITIONAL GUIDELINES

To keep you healthy, you should choose foods that are lower in fat. Remember, I don't want you going overboard with this. I don't want you severely restricting fat grams or calories. You are going to control your eating primarily by limiting portion sizes and eating a specific number of times each day.

Whenever possible choose foods that are lower in fat. Keep in mind, however, that as part of your program (as described in the next chapter) I will be asking you to eat higher-fat foods occasionally in moderation. Flexibility is the key to overcoming the perfectionistic, all-or-nothing thinking that is a major cause of your binge eating.

Here are some guidelines to help you choose lower-fat foods:

1. Drink skim or 1 percent milk
2. Choose low-fat cheese (containing two to three or fewer grams of fat per ounce) and low-fat yogurt
3. Choose meats with less fat such as eye of the

round, top round, sirloin, tenderloin, and T-bone
steak, veal, pork tenderloin

4. Remove skin from poultry
5. Choose low-fat cold cuts
6. Choose fresh or frozen vegetables without sauces
7. Choose fresh fruit, fruit juices, canned fruit in its own juice with no sugar added
8. Choose muffins, biscuits, or rolls with two or fewer grams of fat such as English muffins
9. Choose cereals with two or fewer grams of fat and six or fewer grams of sugar
10. Choose red as opposed to white sauces for pasta and other dishes
11. Eat foods that are baked, broiled, boiled, or roasted as opposed to fried
12. Choose sherbet or sorbet or ice cream with less than five grams of fat per ½ cup serving

Another way to keep fat low in your diet is to plan your seven dinner meals for the week based on the following plan:

Poultry—any two dinners per week
Pasta or vegetable dish—any two dinners per week
Fish or shellfish—any two dinners per week
Lean red meat—one dinner per week

You should be eating a variety of foods, concentrating on lower-fat foods. When confronted with choices, ask yourself which are the unwise, better, and best choices. No matter what you choose, stick to the serving sizes that I have outlined for you.

The success of the Mindful-Eating Program is dependent on your following this flexible dietary plan. This is new to you and you may find yourself resisting at first. Because of the nature of your binge-eating problem you will want more restriction. Just remember that there is structure to the eating plan in terms of regularly scheduled eating times and portion control. Give it a chance and it will work for you.

CHAPTER 12

....

Food Is Not the Enemy: Learning to Eat "Forbidden" Foods

One of the most important elements of your program is to accustom yourself to eating food in moderation. In the last chapter, I discussed portion size guidelines for everyday meals and snacks. Now you are ready to tackle a more difficult challenge—learning to eat "forbidden" foods in moderation.

"Forbidden" foods are those that probably caused you the most difficulty in the past. They are the foods that most diets eliminate from your food plan. They are foods you avoid so you won't binge.

Avoidance of potential binge foods is a main part of your problem. By totally avoiding certain foods, you avoid binge eating for a while, but avoidance is only a temporary solution. Total restriction reinforces all-or-nothing thinking so that when you succumb to the temptation of these foods, you binge. Then you tell yourself that you have "blown your diet" and you feel like a total failure. In the long run, food avoidance does not help you diet and, in fact, makes you more vulnerable to binge eating.

....

WHY YOUR APPROACH TO FOOD
IS LIKE HAVING A PHOBIA

One way to think about your avoidance of certain types of food is to think of yourself as having a phobia. A phobia is an unrealistic fear of a person, object, or situation. People develop unrealistic fears of many things such as heights, open spaces, airplane travel, or spiders. To avoid anxiety associated with these fears, people often avoid contact with these situations or objects. This will work as long as you never come in contact with any of the situations that trigger your phobia.

Let's say you were scared to fly and avoided doing so. If an emergency arose that required you to fly a long distance in an airplane, you would be in big trouble. You would be forced to face up to your fears without preparation. Your experience with flying has been all-or-nothing: total avoidance or total panic. You never learned to confront and overcome your fear.

The most successful way for you to overcome binge eating is the same way you would learn to overcome your fear of flying—one step at a time. Treatment of a phobia requires gradual exposure and experience with the feared situation. The key word is "gradual" because that way you experience success each step of the way and never encounter overwhelming fear. Little by little, you develop more confidence and belief in yourself and in your ability to handle your anxiety. Your gradual behavior change and success experiences have changed your inner thoughts and feelings.

This is an important lesson to learn. We do not have to wait until our feelings, thoughts, and motivations dissipate to change a problem behavior in our lives. Sometimes, the best approach is to modify the behavior first, even though your belief in your ability to change may be weak, with the result that your confidence, belief, and hope increase as a consequence.

The same is true with your eating. Let's suppose that your favorite food is ice cream. You probably would be very skeptical if I told you that in a few weeks you will be able to eat a half cup serving of your favorite ice cream and restrain yourself from eating any more. Your reaction to my prediction might be, "But, Dr. Miller, I have never eaten just one small serving of ice cream in my life. Whenever ice cream is around, particularly chocolate ice cream, I eat the whole carton. I'm ashamed to say it, but I have eaten as much as a quart of ice cream at one sitting. There's no way I could eat just one small bowl. The best way for me to keep from bingeing on ice cream is to avoid it altogether. I'm just too weak."

If that is what you are thinking, you are like most of my clients. But I am going to prove you wrong. I am going to show you that you *can* learn to eat *all* food in moderation without losing control. I don't care how many times you have overindulged in the past or how discouraged you are about your binge eating. All I ask for is your trust and faith.

WHAT ARE YOUR
10 FAVORITE FOODS?

To begin with, I want you to think about your favorite binge foods. These are the foods you avoid when you are dieting.

These are the foods that you fear, the ones that tempt you the most, the ones that produce out-of-control eating. Another way of thinking of this is that these are the foods that control you, that keep you feeling miserable. If you continue to avoid them, they will continue to control you. To be free, you must confront and conquer them.

Before we take on that challenge, let's first find out what your binge foods are. I want you to clear your mind and think about the foods that give you the most trouble. These are the "forbidden" foods. These are the foods you eat when you binge. I realize that you could binge on any food but I am sure you have your favorites. Some people crave candy and chocolate, others, meat and cheese, and still others, bread and butter. It could be anything. A client once told me that she loved to binge on goldfish! I was a bit taken aback by this revelation until I realized that she was talking about cheese-flavored, goldfish-shaped snacks.

On a piece of paper, write a list of 10 of your favorite binge foods. You don't need to be very specific unless you want to be. For example, candy bars would be one item, even though you may enjoy several different types. However, if one type of candy or cheese or snack food is much more appealing to you than others, list it as a separate item. Keep in mind that we are trying to determine the binge potential of these foods. You may have little interest in cheddar cheese but lose control and binge on brie.

Once you have identified your binge foods, rank them in order based on how difficult it would be for you to eat just a little without overeating. The type of food that would be the most difficult for you to resist would be ranked number 1. Number the foods until you get to number 10, the food on your list that would be the easiest to control.

Several years ago I was consulted by Jack, a 42-year-old emergency room physician whose binge eating had resulted in a 40-pound weight gain since he graduated from medical school. His schedule was a hectic one, with days of nonstop emergency care followed by days off when his time was completely his own. Jack was recently divorced and had just moved and taken on a new position with a large teaching hospital. He knew very few people in his new environment and experienced loneliness and depression when he was home alone, away from work. These idle, lonely hours were his high-risk times when he was most likely to binge. I asked Jack to construct a list of binge foods for me and to rank them as I have just described. Here's what his list looked like:

Jack's List of Binge Foods

1. Steak
2. Cheeseburgers
3. French fries
4. Nachos
5. Hot dogs
6. Cheese
7. Bread (Italian or French)
8. Peanut butter
9. Cookies (especially chocolate chip)
10. Potato chips

As you can see, Jack was most tempted by foods that were high in fat, many high in protein and fat such as red meat and cheese. When trying to lose weight (which he had done 12 times in the past six years), Jack chose very restrictive diets and avoided these foods completely. In fact, he preferred liquid formula diets during which he ate only once a day.

His diets would usually last four or five weeks. Then, he would succumb to the temptation of one of his binge foods. During one episode he ordered the following at the window of a fast-food restaurant on his way home from the hospital: three double-bacon cheeseburgers, three extra-large french fries, and a large chocolate milkshake. The server even made the comment, "Taking dinner home to the family?" to which he just nodded and said nothing. His embarrassment made him feel worse about what he was doing but it did not stop him. He rushed home, quickly ate the food, and felt frustrated and upset with himself. His thoughts were, "There I go again. Now I'm off my diet. I'll never be able to lose weight. What's the use? I give up. Why should I even try?"

Fortunately, I was able to help Jack overcome his binge eating and his weight problem. After we normalized his eating schedule with the Mindful Eater's Food Plan, he was ready to battle his binge foods. Even after he compiled his list of binge foods, it took some persuading to convince Jack that this was the proper course of action. After all, he had spent the last several years avoiding the foods that I was now going to suggest that he eat. Once he realized that the process of doing this would be a slow, gradual one in order to maximize success, he agreed to give it a try.

GUIDED EXPOSURE AND RESPONSE PREVENTION

Guided Exposure is a method by which you are gradually confronted with binge foods in moderation with the goal of conditioning you to be able to eat small portions. **Response Prevention** refers to establishing a protected or safe atmosphere for this exposure so that you are prevented from overeating. We can do this in a number of ways, such as ensuring that no more than one portion of the binge food is available or arranging for a supportive friend to be with you at the time.

....

THE FOUR STEPS TO MAKING FRIENDS WITH YOUR BINGE FOODS

Guided Exposure must be accomplished in a systematic and gradually progressive manner. The important goal is to insure success each time you eat a former binge food. That is, we want you to succeed by eating only a portion of the food and no more. Such success builds your confidence and convinces you that you can control your eating. If this training progresses too quickly, you run the risk of falling back into your binge-eating pattern. This would reinforce old habits and discourage you.

The general procedure of Guided Exposure is to schedule times during which you eat a specified portion of one of your binge foods. These times should occur on a regular weekly basis so that eating moderate portions of binge foods becomes part of your regular diet.

Here's how to proceed.

STEP 1: HOW TO CHOOSE WHAT TO EAT

Start with binge food number 10 on your binge list. Of all of the listed binge foods, this one should be the easiest for you to control. As you succeed with each food on your list, you will be moving gradually up from binge food number 10 to binge food number 1. You should wait until you have eaten a binge food twice in moderation before you proceed up the list. If, after two separate practice sessions, you still feel uneasy or anxious about the eating experience, practice with the same food until you feel more comfortable. After you are able to eat a portion of two or three binge foods without overeating, your confidence in your ability to control your eating will increase quickly and dramatically.

STEP 2: WHEN TO EAT YOUR BINGE FOODS

Schedule *two times in the next few days* when you will eat a portion of the binge food that you have chosen. *This eating should be part of one of your regularly scheduled meals or snacks.* This is extremely important since I want you to discontinue all unscheduled eating. Eating, even binge food, is okay but only at times when you have scheduled a meal or snack. For example, if the binge food is a candy bar, it could be included as a dinnertime dessert or as a mid-afternoon snack. These practice sessions should be scheduled two times a week. Guided Exposure sessions can occur at home, at a restaurant, or at a friend's home.

For example, if you have been invited out to dinner at someone's home and dessert will probably be served, this would be a good opportunity for you to plan to eat one serving of dessert.

STEP 3: HOW MUCH OF YOUR BINGE FOOD TO EAT

The next question you might have is, "How do I determine a portion size?" You can do this in a couple of ways. First, if the food chosen is a packaged food such as potato chips or ice cream, the package label will tell you what portion is considered to be one serving size. You may be surprised by what you find. For example, if you check the label, you'll find that 14 potato chips constitute one serving. Did you know that a pint of ice cream contains four servings? That's right. A standard serving of ice cream is half a cup.

To give you an idea of what I am talking about, here is a sampling of some common binge foods and their serving sizes.

Binge Food Serving Sizes

Cookies 3
Large cookies..1
Doughnuts 1
Cheez-It crackers 27
Goldfish crackers......................................52
Candy bar..1 medium

M&Ms ....¼ cup
Wheat crackers.......................................5

When in doubt, use your judgment depending on the size of the item. If certain doughnuts are very small, two or three may be more appropriate than one. However, because of your binge history you might want to check the serving size with a couple of friends to see if they would consider it an average portion.

STEP 4: HOW YOU CAN INSURE SUCCESS

Only schedule Guided Exposure sessions on days when you are feeling calm and self-assured. Do not schedule a binge food eating practice on days when you are tense, angry, depressed, or otherwise emotionally upset. Also, do not schedule one of these sessions on a day when you are having strong cravings to binge. If the session has already been scheduled and something comes up that day to upset you, cancel the session and reschedule it for the next day or the day after.

It is very important to make certain that only one portion of your binge food is available to you, especially when you first begin your Guided Exposure sessions. In order to do this, you could arrange these sessions to occur when you are eating in a restaurant or when you have been invited to someone's home for lunch or dinner. If you are going to eat your binge food at home, buy only the portion needed for your session. If this is not possible due to the container or package, arrange to have family members or friends (invite others to lunch or dinner that day) eat the same food with you so that there is none left over. If no other solution is available, you may have to take one portion and throw out the rest. This may sound wasteful but you must do whatever it takes not to have tempting leftovers available to you.

STEP 5: HOW YOU SHOULD EAT YOUR BINGE FOODS

It is extremely important to allow enough time during these sessions to eat your food slowly and mindfully. That is why you should never plan a Guided Exposure session when you are in a hurry or upset. You should take your time and keep your mind on the process of eating.

As I discussed in Chapter 9, you should practice Mindful-Eating Awareness whenever you eat. This is especially true when you are trying to accustom yourself to eating binge foods in moderation. During your past binge episodes you ate rapidly and with little or no awareness. To change the pattern, you must change these two aspects of eating. This will be a new experience for you and a little difficult at first. You must concentrate on eating slowly and paying detailed attention to what you are doing. Remember the Raisin Meditation I described in Chapter 9. You must pay attention to the look of the food, its texture, its taste, and what you are thinking and feeling as you are eating it. If you are eating with others, try to take twice as long to eat your binge food as anyone else.

When you are finished eating, evaluate how you did. During the first few sessions, you may find that your mind wanders a bit or even that you fall back into your old pattern of mindlessness. Do not allow your mind to go blank. Stay attentive and aware. If you have trouble with a wavering attention span during the first session or two, don't worry about it. You will improve with time and practice.

THE CASE OF ANNIE

One of my most successful clients was Annie, a 57-year-old artist and the mother of two grown children. The Guided Exposure phase of my program had a particularly significant impact on Annie's progress in freeing herself from her dependence on food.

Throughout her life, Annie always had a tendency to be overweight. She remembers going with her mother to a local diet program when she was only 14 years of age. As an adult, she had tried just about every diet and weight-loss program available. She would typically lose some or all of her weight but would eventually gain it all back.

At age 57, her weight of 205 pounds was higher than it had ever been. When she came to see me for the first time she had not dieted for two years. She was so frustrated with her past failures that she simply had stopped trying to lose weight. She felt that her eating was totally out of control but she just did not care anymore. She was frustrated and depressed. She hated the way she looked. Her way of handling her misery was avoidance. She just stopped thinking about her eating and her weight.

Annie had not weighed herself in six months. She would not think about or talk about her weight. She would walk away when her husband or children tried to discuss their concern about her weight and her health. "Leave me alone. I don't want to talk about it," she would say.

Annie was also becoming much less interested in her artistic pursuits. She had been an accomplished children's portrait painter but had not taken on a commission for quite a long time. She had lost passion for her work as well as confidence in her abilities. She was depressed and feeling quite worthless. She had little interest in friends or activities out of the house.

My evaluation of Annie revealed that she had a major binge-eating problem that was getting worse. Binge eating had been the culprit in causing her to regain weight she had lost on diets over her lifetime. While Annie realized that she suffered from compulsive overeating, she thought of this behavior as a character defect as opposed to a clinical problem that required specialized treatment. She had always thought that if she dieted long enough she could overcome her eating difficulties.

After explaining the nature of her binge-eating disorder and how we were going to overcome it, I started Annie out with a scheduled eating plan such as the one I described in Chapter 11. Next, I described Guided Exposure and how we were going to help her learn to eat small to moderate amounts of her binge foods. Annie resisted at first, saying, "You don't understand; I think I'm addicted to food. I know I don't have the willpower it takes to eat a small portion of chocolate." She was so anxious about Guided Exposure that she wanted to eliminate it from the program. She promised to follow all of my other advice except for this. She insisted that, in her case, it would be better to avoid these foods forever.

I pointed out to Annie that she had tried the all-or-nothing approach all of her life and it had failed repeatedly. After much discussion, she finally agreed to give it a try. She wrote a list of her binge foods and rank ordered them as follows:

Annie's List of Binge Foods

1. Brownies
2. Boxed candy
3. Candy bars
4. Ice cream
5. Jelly doughnuts
6. Cheesecake
7. Oreo cookies
8. Peanuts or cashews
9. Snack crackers
10. Pizza

We then determined what portion of each food would be considered a serving size. We agreed on these portion sizes: 1 brownie, 3 pieces of candy from a box, 1 medium candy bar (1 oz. size), ½ cup of ice cream, 1 jelly doughnut, 1 slice of cheesecake, 3 Oreo cookies, a palmful of nuts, 1 small package of snack crackers, and 2 slices of pizza.

We began Annie's practice sessions with pizza since it was the lowest on her list, the binge food she considered to be the easiest to control. She had been following a scheduled eating plan of healthy foods for two weeks, avoiding all binge foods on her list. She decided that on Wednesday night she and her husband would go to a pizzeria for dinner. This worked out well since she could order pizza by the slice. The individual slices were quite large so she decided to order one slice of pizza topped with vegetables and a small salad. Her husband, who was naturally slim and could always eat without gaining weight (an occasional source of intense frustration for Annie), ordered three slices for himself.

Annie was a bit anxious since she felt guilty about eating pizza while she was trying to control her eating. This was a totally new experience for her. Her guilt subsided when she realized that I had prescribed pizza for her. In fact, I told her that once she scheduled a binge food practice session, she should eat her portion of food whether she wanted it or not.

She ate her pizza slowly and deliberately and enjoyed each mouthful. She ate slowly enough so that even though her husband ordered three times as much pizza, they finished eating at about the same time. Momentarily, Annie thought that another slice of pizza would taste good. She was no longer hungry but neither was she totally full. However, she remained strong and did not order any more food. It helped to have her husband with her.

For the next pizza practice session Annie and her husband ordered a medium-sized pizza to be delivered at home. Annie planned to eat two slices, which she did. Her husband had four slices. Annie ate her pizza slowly and mindfully and enjoyed it. She felt satisfied and did not have the urge to eat any more, in spite of the fact that two slices of pizza were left.

Now the question became what to do with the remaining two slices that neither wanted. Annie and I actually had discussed a plan should this situation arise. While Annie did not crave more pizza at that moment, what was going to happen later that evening if two slices were still available? Remember, the goal of Guided Exposure is to eat a portion of a binge food and *prevent* further eating. The best way to prevent eating is to eliminate the binge food from your surroundings, once a portion has been consumed.

Annie, with the consent and understanding of her husband, decided to throw the remaining pizza away. In fact, she broke it up and put it in the garbage disposal. This may seem like a waste of food but you must remember that it is essential to take whatever action is necessary to prevent overeating. You probably will not have to do this forever. However, it will never be a good idea for you to keep a lot of tempting food around the house. Would a recovering alcoholic keep the house stocked with liquor?

As Annie progressed through her list she developed more and more confidence in herself. She did have two slips along the way, which were probably due to her trying to advance up her binge food list too quickly. One slip occurred when she reached food item number 3. She bought one candy bar at the grocery store. It was 4:00 and time for her afternoon snack. She was a bit rushed that day so instead of going home to eat the candy bar she ate it in the car in the parking lot of the grocery store. She was also a bit discouraged that day. She had lost weight each week for the past four weeks but at her weigh-in that morning, the scale had not changed. Temporary plateaus are a natural part of the weight-loss process but can be frustrating.

Annie ate the candy bar, but much faster than she should have. Her mind was wandering and she was having difficulty staying focused and mindful. The candy tasted very, very good and was soothing and calming her. Impulsively and without much thought, she went back into the store and bought two more candy bars. Once back in the car, she ate them very quickly. Afterward, she felt very guilty and angry with herself. She had let her guard down and her binge behavior had returned.

Fortunately, I had warned Annie that this might happen. It is perfectly normal. You should not expect progress to be smooth. A slip does not indicate that you have failed or that you are reverting to your old behavior. It does not mean you are weak or that you have lost your willpower.

Annie was able to put a stop to her old negative thinking about her binge and forgive herself. She realized that she should not have eaten the candy bar in the car and that because she was feeling frustrated, she should have rescheduled her binge food session.

After slowly working up her binge food list, Annie developed more and more confidence. She could not believe that she was actually eating portions of food that had controlled her in the past. She was eating on a schedule and had only binged two times in the past two months. This was a dramatic change since she had been bingeing three times a week when she first came to see me.

Annie put her experience this way:

I finally realized that food is not the enemy. The enemy was within me. I took control of my eating and of my life. I feel stronger now than I ever have. Because of the Guided Exposure I have proven to myself that I can control my eating. I never thought it was possible.

Two years after beginning this program, Annie is a new person. She gradually lost 55 pounds and has overcome her binge-eating problem. In the two years, she binged on only two occasions, after the death of her mother and during a time when one of her children was having emotional problems. She is no longer depressed and feels exuberant about life. Soon after she began to feel more confident about her eating, she resumed her painting. She rediscovered her passion for art and now has a 12-month waiting list of portrait commissions.

....

A WORD ABOUT YOUR ATTITUDE

I want to say again that I realize that confronting your binge foods in this manner is foreign to you. In fact, it is not just unfamiliar territory, it goes against what you think is right for you. Because of your all-or-nothing approach to dieting, avoidance of binge foods would be more natural for you than scheduling yourself to eat them from time to time.

Because of this, just like Annie, you may resist what I am asking you to do. Many of my clients feel very anxious when they first try to eat binge foods in small doses. This tension is temporary. The payoff is enormous. Not only do you control your binge eating and lose weight, but you change your life in the process.

In addition to changing your binge-eating behavior directly through Guided Exposure, we also must begin a process of mental and emotional changes that are related to your binge eating. In the next two chapters, I will show you how to gain control over your emotional life and keep a positive, in-control attitude.

CHAPTER 13

....

Mindfulness Over Emotional Eating

Sally is a 35-year-old office manager living in New York City. She has fought a battle with her weight ever since she can remember. When I first evaluated her several years ago she was 65 pounds overweight and extremely distressed by her weight and binge eating. A promotion at work that added more responsibility, higher expectations, and longer hours had resulted in a worsening of her binge-eating problem. Although she enjoyed her work, it took a lot out of her. She was efficient and well organized and took pride in being a bit on the perfectionistic side. Sally set very high standards for herself and was determined to take advantage of her promotion to advance her career. Her new boss was very demanding and extremely critical. To add to her stress, some of the employees whom she was now supervising had resented her being promoted ahead of them. The office environment was quite tense.

Up until the time of her promotion, Sally had at

least been maintaining her weight and was only bingeing occasionally. Now she binged almost every day. Sally lived alone in a small Manhattan apartment. Lately, she would arrive home at about 7:00 P.M., hungry, exhausted, and totally stressed out. She often skipped lunch to save on calories and to keep up with her work. Her typical routine was to fix herself a glass of wine and collapse on her couch in front of the television. One glass usually led to two and sometimes three. Sally began every evening with the solemn vow that she would have just one glass of wine, followed by a salad and a healthy frozen meal. Her freezer was always stocked with a plentiful supply of low-calorie, low-fat packaged frozen meals.

Her strong resolve almost always fell short. Her emotions seemed to take control of her intellect. Hunger, anger, loneliness, and fatigue overwhelmed her. Often her thoughts were, "I worked hard all day. I deserve a treat. I'm too tired to eat right. Besides, I did everything I was supposed to do today. Now I want to do what *I* want to do. I'll get back on my diet tomorrow." With that, Sally would telephone for a delivery of spareribs or Chinese food. Hesitantly, she admitted to me that she typically ordered two whole meals, even pretending in her conversations with take-out restaurants that someone else was with her. She would order one meal, then say to her phantom friend, "Oh, and what will you have?" and then order a different second meal.

On one occasion, after bingeing at 8:00 P.M. on two portions of lasagna, she called another Italian restaurant for a delivery of six cannoli and a bottle of wine. When ordering, she explained that she was having friends over for refreshments after the theater. She hated herself for lying, but she was so self-conscious and embarrassed about binge eating that she became unrealistically desperate to keep it a secret.

Sally's case is very typical. Emotional stress is the major cause of binge eating. It is the number one circumstance that triggers most episodes of overindulgence with food among binge eaters. What emotions trigger your food cravings? When I pose this question to my clients, I hear a long list of negative emotions including tension, anxiety, depression, anger, boredom, restlessness, resentment, feeling overwhelmed, feeling misunderstood, and loneliness. We eat for a variety of emotional reasons. We overeat for comfort and self-gratification. We overeat for reward. We overeat to escape. We even overeat to rebel.

THE NUMBER ONE REASON
FOR BINGE EATING

Emotional distress is the most frequently cited reason for what triggers an episode of binge eating. The most typical emotions associated with bingeing are anxiety, frustration, anger, depression, and loneliness. In studies conducted by myself and colleagues in the Department of Health Promotion and Education at the University of South Carolina, women have a greater problem with emotional eating than do men. They have less confidence than men in their ability to restrain their appetites when they are upset. After the binge is over, women also experience more guilt and depression than men do.

Why Emotions Cause Binge Eating

In Chapter 5, I discussed mood and personality as they relate to the development of binge eating. Let's talk a little more about why emotions and food have become so connected in your life.

It is obvious that food has many meanings in our society. We grow up learning that food is a lot more than nutrition. Food is love, affection, and friendship. When people get together for whatever reason, food is usually involved. Would you ever invite a group of people to your house and not serve something to eat or drink? It might only be a cup of coffee, but it would be a rare event for food to be missing.

When the host or hostess of a dinner party offers you a special homemade dessert, how do you react? Many people tell me that this situation is difficult because they feel it would be rude to refuse. They view the dessert as a gesture of caring, as if a gift were being offered.

The experience of food as comfort goes back to childhood. Many years ago I conducted a study of young children, ages 4 and 5. I wanted to find out whether children this young thought of food as comfort and as a way of coping with emotional distress. I first asked them to pretend they were feeling different emotions. We began with sadness, then went to anger, then boredom, and finally, loneliness. As the children thought about each emotion, I presented them with a series of choices in the form of pictures. For each separate emotion, I asked them, "Which of these would make you feel better if you really had this feeling?" The choices included talking to someone, being hugged or comforted by a parent, being given a new toy or game, playing a game, playing with friends, or eating a favorite food.

The emotion with the greatest connection to eating turned out to be anger. The majority of children chose "eating a favorite food" as their top choice if they were angry at someone or something.

I also asked the children to imagine that each of their parents were experiencing these emotions. The choices were more adult in nature but the question was the same: "Which of these would make your mommy (daddy) feel better if she (he) really had this feeling?" Again, the connection between eating and anger was the strongest of all the emotions. The children chose "eating" and "smoking" as the two top choices to calm an angry mother. The top choices for fathers were "drinking an alcoholic beverage" and "sports or recreational activities."

Even as young as age 4, children are perceiving food as a way to relieve emotion, not only in themselves but in their parents. Of course, seeing what parents do is the way they learn. If Mommy eats when she is upset, that must be the way to feel better emotionally.

Eating under conditions of stress provides a temporary distraction from the problems of life. Eating also reduces tension and provides a feeling of calmness. This is partly psychological and, depending on the type of food eaten, partly physiological. Carbohydrate foods in the form of sweets or starches cause your brain to produce serotonin. This brain chemical makes you feel calm, soothed, relaxed, and a bit drowsy. Certain foods act like tranquilizers in your system.

There is also a relationship between emotional eating and self-esteem. As a binge eater, you are likely to have high expectations of yourself. Many binge eaters are also people-pleasers. Together with a low self-esteem, these qualities result in frequent anxiety or depression caused by worry over letting someone down, performing inadequately, or not living up to your own or others' expectations. Eating serves as a distraction and escape from these negative thoughts about yourself. This explains the "spaced-out," robotlike experiences that occur during a binge. Your mind needs protection against your own derogatory, fault-finding thoughts that make you feel worthless.

MINDFULNESS AND EMOTIONAL CONTROL

Since binge eating, at least in the short-term, helps to calm and distract you when you are upset, we cannot simply take this behavior away without providing other ways for you to deal with stress. From a mind-fulness perspective, there are five ways to gain control over emotions. You can:

1. Be more aware of them
2. Release them
3. Confront them
4. Solve the problems that cause them
5. Let them go

BECOMING MORE AWARE OF EMOTIONS

Becoming more aware of emotions is essential if you ever hope to break the connection between emotions and binge eating. Some binge eaters are blindsided by their emotions and are out of control with their eating before they know it. They often don't realize that they are stressed out until they overeat. Your goal is to be so aware of your feelings that you recognize seeds of resentment or frustration as early as possible on a day-to-day basis. In that way, you can take action before the emotion overwhelms you and leads to binge eating.

To accomplish this goal you must first put yourself into a state of mindfulness when negative feelings occur. This allows you to slow things down, to fight your old style of impulsively reaching for food. Emotions serve as a driving force toward binge eating. Your mind's first instinct is to "go blank" and to pay less attention to feelings and more attention to food. We must break this pattern through mindfulness.

The first step is to find a quiet place that is away from everyone else. Sit in a relaxed but upright position with your feet flat on the floor. Close your eyes, take a deep breath, and slowly let it out. Let go of the recent past and forget about what might be happening in the next few moments. The most important thing for you to do is to concentrate on the present moment, on your present feelings. Right now, what caused those feelings does not matter as much as what the feelings are.

With a sense of alertness and awareness, concentrate on the present moment. Do not try to consciously think of anything. Pay attention to what feelings are in your body. You may be having thoughts as well as feelings but, for now, I just want you to focus on the feelings. You are an observer looking in at yourself. I don't want you to judge your feelings, I simply want you to observe and identify them.

What emotions are inside of you? Are you lonely? Are you afraid? Do you feel panic? Are you mad? Are you sad? Let whatever feelings you have show themselves.

This is an important exercise because some emotions disguise themselves. Under these conditions, it is difficult for us to know exactly what we are feeling or what we can do about it. For example, there is a connection between the emotions of anger and depression. Anger that is turned inward against yourself is frequently felt as depression. You feel sad but you are really mad. Mad at yourself or mad at someone or something else.

It is important to know which emotion is driving your binge eating so you can ask the question, "What do I really want or need right now?" If you are sad you may need comforting, but if you are mad you may need to acknowledge and release the anger or confront the cause of your anger.

RELEASING AND QUIETING EMOTIONS

Once you have acknowledged and identified your feelings, it is important to release or quiet them. Feelings that are kept bottled up get stronger and become much more difficult to control. Feelings can be released in several ways. Probably the best way is to talk or write your feelings out. If you are a private person who does not share feelings easily, this may be difficult for you. You can begin by writing your feelings. Write down whatever you are feeling regardless of what it is. Don't judge it, just observe it and write it down.

Talking about your feelings to a loved one, a friend, or a therapist is even better. When you are releasing feelings, you need a caring, empathetic listener. In trying to help, those close to you may not merely listen but also offer useful advice. This is fine as long as you have had sufficient time to express your emotions. Your main focus should be on releasing and then as a result quieting your thoughts and feelings.

Another great way to release feelings is through physical activity. This can be in the form of exercise such as a walk, swim, bicycle ride, or aerobics class. It might also take the form of a recreational activity or hobby that is physically demanding. Exercise actually releases some of the same brain chemicals that food does, resulting in the production of natural tranquilizers to calm you.

Some emotions need quieting as well as releasing. If you are very tense and nervous, you may need physical relaxation in order to quiet the symptoms of stress in your body. When we are stressed, heart rate increases, breathing becomes shallow and erratic, blood pressure goes up, and muscles tighten.

Mindful meditation is a great way to put your body into a relaxed, slow-motion mode. Meditation that is used for relaxation often focuses on breathing. By controlling and slowing your breathing, you reduce heart rate, blood pressure, respiratory rate, and muscle tension.

The most soothing meditational breathing is known as diaphragm or belly breathing. During this type of breathing your stomach gently rises and then falls with each breath. It rises as you inhale and falls as you exhale. We are born breathing this way but lose touch with it as we become less mindful of the way we breathe. Watch a sleeping baby breathe and you will see what I mean. You'll see a stomach that is gently rising and falling, and a breathing pattern that follows a gentle rhythm.

To quiet and soothe your emotions using belly breathing, find an out-of-the-way place that is free of distractions. Just as I suggested when you were identifying your emotions, sit in a relaxed but upright position. If you are slouched in a chair you will not be able to experience the correct breathing style. A lying position will also work.

Place your palms flat against your stomach. Relax your muscles, particularly those in your stomach. Relax your body. Let your muscles feel relaxed, warm, and heavy. Breathe naturally. Your breathing should be slow and steady. As you breathe, adopt a mindful attitude—pay attention, be aware, focus on the present moment; be an observer, not a judge.

Concentrate exclusively on your breathing. With each breath, focus on your stomach as it gently rises when you inhale and falls when you exhale. Feel your stomach rise and fall against the palms of your hands. Be patient. Do not try to rush. Let your breathing become free and natural. Slow and steady breathing should be your goal. Allow your breathing to slow down.

As you practice belly breathing, you will gradually notice that your breathing will become slow and rhythmical. Your heart rate will become slow and steady. The muscles in your body will feel heavy and warm. Everything in your body will go into slow motion.

Pay attention and be aware of your breathing. If you are distracted by stressful thoughts, be aware of them but *do not* be carried away by them. Acknowledge them but do not let them take your attention away. Bring your attention and concentration back to your breathing. Focus on your stomach as it rises and falls with each breath. The rising and falling of your stomach will keep you centered and keep you calm.

Be careful of distracting thoughts such as, "I'm so upset. I've got a million things to do and I'm sitting here thinking about breathing. I'm wasting time. I have all kinds of problems I should be trying to solve." You can solve your problems later. Right now, your goal is to quiet your emotions so you'll either be able to solve your problem or, if it is not solvable, you'll be able to cope with it better.

You can practice mindful meditation for as long as you want. However, I would suggest a minimum of 15 to 20 minutes at a time. Keep doing it until you feel more relaxed, calm, and peaceful.

CONFRONTING EMOTIONS

You should confront your emotions when you have negative feelings that will not go away. There are times when we become upset and, in spite of our best efforts, we remain upset over an extended period of time. You might brood over something that is making you angry, frustrated, or depressed. When this happens, you may have to confront your feelings more directly. Distraction may not be effective because the negative feeling that keeps returning is very strong and overpowering.

Mindfulness provides an excellent way to confront your feelings. When you develop a mindful attitude you can come face-to-face with frustration, fear, anger, or depression and overpower them. To be mindful is to be an observer of feelings, not a judge.

Anger is an emotion that often triggers binge eating. Mindfulness can allow you to experience anger without judging it. You will be able to look at anger and to acknowledge it. You will find that you can come face-to-face with it. You'll be amazed to discover that the more you are able to confront your anger, the stronger and less angry you will feel.

Kate was extremely frustrated by her elderly mother, who was very demanding and critical of her. No matter how much Kate did for her, Kate's mother had the habit of making her feel guilty. In fact, the more Kate did to help her, the more her mother demanded. What made matters worse is that her mother would compare Kate to her brothers, saying, "Your brothers are always so considerate. They both sent flowers for Mother's Day. I wish you were more like them." The truth of the matter was that Kate's brothers rarely visited their mother or did anything for her. The bulk of the responsibility for care was left up to Kate.

Understandably, Kate remained in a constant state of frustration over this situation. She felt her mother was being unrealistic, unfair, and manipulative. She could not get over her anger at her brothers, who would not help, even when she asked or demanded they do so. Talking to her husband about her feelings helped some, but she continued to brood about the unfairness of her situation. She tried to relax and meditate but the feelings of anger overpowered her. Since these emotions were interfering with her progress in overcoming her binge eating, I convinced Kate to try to confront her anger through mindfulness.

She began to practice confrontational mindfulness daily. I suggested that she establish a regular 20-minute period each day for this activity. She worked on developing a mindful attitude of nonjudgmental awareness during these times. Focusing on the present moment and blocking out the past and future, Kate concentrated on her feelings of anger and resentment. She found this difficult at first. When she thought about her anger, it seemed to intensify. She felt more anger. The trouble was that Kate was not maintaining a mindful attitude during these times. She was judging. When she felt her anger, her thoughts would get out of control. She thought, "This is not fair. Why do I have to do all the work? I love my mother, but she frustrates me so much. I am mad at her but I feel guilty for my feelings." These are judgmental thoughts, not mindful thoughts. When these thoughts occurred, I encouraged Kate to be aware of them, to acknowledge them, but to let them go.

It may sound odd or simpleminded to you that emotions lose their power when we simply look at and confront them in an aware, nonjudgmental way. I can assure you that it happens. When it does happen, you not only feel better emotionally, but you feel a sense of emotional freedom and personal control of your life that is exhilarating. In Kate's case, she gradually stopped binge eating, lost weight, and took charge of her life. Her mother did not change, her brothers continued to refuse to help, but she was free from the emotions that were keeping her dependent on binge eating.

SOLVING PROBLEMS THAT CAUSE EMOTIONS

There are some stresses in life that require action and problem solving. We all know that problems are a normal part of life whether we like it or not. We also know that we can learn ways to cope with everyday problems. This involves being aware of what is causing us stress and evaluating various courses of action that might reduce our stress. You are doing something about your binge-eating problem by reading this book and putting my program into action. You may not have known what course of action to take to solve your problem but you sought professional advice and found it. This is how you must approach other problems in your life.

Problem solving as a solution to stress requires a take-charge attitude. I have found that many of my clients have this attitude when it comes to business or family obligations. They identify problems, decide on a course of action, and take whatever actions are needed to resolve the issue. But because of low self-esteem combined with a desire to please others, my clients feel very inhibited and insecure when it comes to problems related to their personal lives. People problems, emotional problems, and food problems seem beyond their comprehension or control.

You must begin to change that. You must take charge of your personal and emotional life as well. You can do it. You have what it takes. Your binge eating has probably gotten you down so much that you've lost confidence in yourself. I would like to give that confidence back to you.

The first step in changing a problem is to define it in very precise terms. Sometimes problems seem overwhelming because we fail to see the exact nature of what is involved. Let's suppose you tell me, "I am frustrated and upset because my husband and I don't get along." Or, "I resent my job and that causes me to eat." So you stay frustrated and upset and resentful, waiting for your husband or your job to change for the better. Because these problems are defined in such vague terms, no useful solutions seem possible.

You must redefine the problem in more specific terms if you are going to come up with solutions. Spend some time thinking about these problems. Be much more specific about what is going on that is upsetting you. What do you mean when you say you and your husband do not get along? What about your job do you resent? You don't need to look for reasons. Just describe the problems in a more detailed way. For example, in thinking of your marriage, you might say, "When I talk to my husband about my feelings, he doesn't listen. He jumps to conclusions, gives me quick advice on what to do, but doesn't allow me to get out my frustrations. And he never talks to me about how he is feeling. I know he is under a lot of pressure at work but he never talks about it. This makes me feel isolated and alone."

Your job stress might be redefined as, "I work in my family's business and my hours are long. I am a perfectionist in my work but I can't seem to get the rest of my family to do things the way I think they should be done. I am doing more than everyone else and I don't even have time to eat lunch. I want to exercise to help lose weight but I'm so tired at the end of the day, I just collapse when I get home." Now the problem becomes more detailed and possible solutions can be formulated.

The next question to ask about any stress in your life is, "What must happen so that this situation is no longer a problem?" You must now think about possible solutions. To maximize the chances of finding a successful one, you must brainstorm as many alternatives as possible. Brainstorming is a method by which you think of every possible alternative, whether it makes sense or not. It is important to write these possible solutions in a notebook or on a piece of paper. Don't discount any of them even if they seem silly or unrealistic at first. Write down every alternative that comes into your mind.

Next, look at all the solutions and think about the potential consequences of each course of action. If it helps, rate each solution using the following rating scale.

++ Very good
 + Good
 0 Neutral
 - Bad
-- Very bad

Consider the *Very good* solutions and decide which has the best chance of success. Remember, in life, most solutions are less than perfect. There may always be some doubt in your mind about the best possibility.

The final stage of problem solving requires you to implement the solution. In the job stress case, it might obligate you to talk to the other family members at work about reducing your time or effort in the business. It might involve asking for or even demanding help so that you have time for lunch and so that you can finish early enough in the day to schedule your exercise.

I realize that life's problems are not simple and do not always follow a neatly packaged, step-by-step format. Sometimes you know the correct solution but you have trouble implementing it. You might feel guilty making demands on your family at work. You might lack the necessary assertiveness to stand up for yourself. In these cases you might need support from friends, relatives, or a therapist to help you follow the necessary course of action. Otherwise, you may continue to feel stressed and overwhelmed and continue to binge.

LETTING GO OF EMOTIONS

Sometimes an emotion or thoughts about a problem may keep bothering you no matter what you do. You may not be able to get it out of your mind. You may think about the problem and feel upset about it all the time. You may brood about it.

You will be left with anxiety, anger, or frustration

when a problem is over but you still have not completely resolved it in your mind. You will also suffer
continued emotional distress over problems that will
not go away—ones in which there does not seem to
be a ready solution.

Under these conditions, the solution to controlling your emotions is simply to *let them go*. I know
this sounds easier said than done, but let me tell you
a story that illustrates what I am talking about. This
story is often told when teaching novices the funda-
mentals of mindfulness and meditation.

In India, monkeys are captured in an unusual way.
The hunters cut a hole in a coconut and scoop out
the inside. They make the hole big enough for a
monkey's hand to fit through. Two small holes are
then drilled into the opposite end of the coconut so
that it can be tied to a tree. Next a banana is placed
inside the coconut. The hunters then hide to wait for
the monkeys to arrive. Each monkey, tempted by the
banana, places his hand into the hole in the coconut
and grabs the fruit. Unfortunately for the monkey,
the hole is designed in such a way that an open hand
can move freely in and out but a closed fist will be
too big. The hunters reappear and capture the monkey since it is trapped by not being able to remove its
clenched fist from the coconut. All the monkey has
to do to achieve freedom is to let go of the banana
and remove its hand. The monkeys never do it. They
are always captured.

When your anxiety, resentment, or frustration over
a problem in your life continues, you must consider

letting go of the banana. Your natural instinct may be to hold the banana tighter and tighter but the end result is that you are a captive of your own emotions.

A mindful attitude can help you let go. Close your eyes, clear your mind, and get into a mindful state. Close off the past and future. Focus only on this moment in time. Pay attention and stay aware. Most important, as I have said before, be an observer, not a judge. Concentrate on the emotion that is bothering you. As an observer and not a judge, you must remember that feelings and thoughts are neither "good" nor "bad." They exist. If you are feeling resentful, do not label or judge it. Simply be aware of it.

Separate your resentment from yourself. Look at it objectively, as an observer would. You are not your thoughts and feelings. They are not part of you. They do not define you. When you say, "I am very angry and resentful," you are giving in to the notion that anger is part of who you are. When you think this way, you will feel overwhelmed by your emotions. You will feel controlled by them because you see them as an appendage, just like an arm or a leg. If you *are* your anger, it will always be with you. You will not be able to get rid of it.

By letting go of your resentment, you are disowning it. You are saying that it is no longer a part of you. You are substituting "I am very angry" with "I am having angry thoughts and feelings." In this way, you are acknowledging anger as a state of mind. Anger is nothing more than what you are saying to yourself and what you are feeling at this moment in time. It is temporary. It comes and goes. Because of this, you can open up your hand, just like the monkeys in India could, and let go of your resentments. Negative thoughts and feelings are totally within your control. You can allow them to stay within you, poisoning your mind, body, and spirit, or you can choose to release them.

Letting go is not easy and you have to work on it. With time, and continually practicing a mindful attitude, you will learn to let go. It doesn't take a lot of effort. It only involves opening up your closed fist and letting go. Afterward, you will experience a feeling of emotional relief and peace of spirit that will be exhilarating.

CHAPTER 14

························

Changing Your Perfectionistic Ways: Mindful Mind Control

One of the most typical characteristics of binge eaters is a particular way of looking at the world known as dichotomous, all-or-nothing thinking. Binge eaters interpret events in their lives in perfectionistic, rigid, black-and-white terms. When this thinking style is applied to eating and weight control it becomes one of the major contributors to binge-eating problems.

Nicholas was a successful insurance salesman working for a large agency in Atlanta. The problem of being overweight ran in his family. Both parents, his brother, and his sister were all obese. He had fought a battle with his weight since childhood. At age 38, when he first came to see me about his binge eating, he weighed 50 pounds more than he should.

Nicholas was a veteran dieter and had tried everything from Weight Watchers and diet books to diet pills, hypnosis, and acupuncture. He was an on-again, off-again dieter. Diets would begin well. He followed the plan, lost weight, and began to feel good about himself. After a week or two, Nicholas's hunger would get the best of him. He did not crave specific foods such as sweets or cheese or bread. When dieting, he experienced a great deal of hunger, which he found difficult to control. He put it this way:

I love to eat. It's one of my favorite things to do. And, when I eat, I eat a lot. I eat huge portions and never am satisfied. When I'm dieting, I feel hungry and deprived most of the time. I think about food and eating all the time.

Once he overate on his diet, Nicholas was defeated. He felt so guilty about "breaking" the diet, he gave up. His guilt drove him to continue eating until he felt totally out of control. During these times his thoughts went something like this:

There I go again. After only a week, I'm off my diet. I failed again. I'll never be able to lose weight. I must be addicted to food. What's the use? This just proves I don't have any willpower.

Interestingly enough, although Nicholas was perfectionistic in other areas of life, he did not react in this same defeatist way when faced with adversity in those other areas. This is typical of most of my clients. Because of this, I usually take the opportunity to ask, "Do you ever make mistakes in other areas of your life?" "Of course," they reply. I then ask them to tell me what happens when they make these mistakes, what they usually say to themselves. Here's how Nicholas answered when I inquired about mistakes at work:

> Well, I usually just try harder. I set very high standards for my sales performance and I usually meet my goals. Sometimes I screw up and lose a sale or make some stupid mistake when I bid for the business. I just figure that's part of life and try to be more careful the next time. There's always another day and another potential customer.

"So," I replied, "you give up the battle and think of yourself as a failure when you make a dietary mistake but you try harder and search out new opportunities when you fall short with insurance sales?" Clients seem surprised by this obvious discrepancy in their ways of thinking about situations related to dieting and those related to other aspects of their lives. Think about this in your own case. If you can think more positively about nondieting "failures," you can certainly learn to put these same thought patterns into practice with food and eating. But somehow, normal mistakes with dieting are viewed as character flaws while other mistakes are just temporary setbacks.

Here's some diet logic for you to think about:

Diet Logic

1. Human beings on diets goof up from time to time
2. I am a human being
3. Therefore, I should goof up from time to time

Because of all-or-nothing thinking, you may be just like Nicholas, living his life either "on" or "off" a diet. His perfectionistic nature caused him to set very high standards for himself. These standards became obvious when I asked him to tell me what his expectations were whenever he started a new diet. He replied, "I expect that this will be my very last diet. I feel that I should exercise every day, without fail, for the rest of my life. I also expect to avoid eating all high-fat, high-calorie foods and to eat small-to-moderate-size portions of every food I eat. By doing this, I expect to lose 50 pounds in two months and never gain back even one pound of it."

Nicholas had convinced himself that these were realistic, attainable goals. To him, being less than perfect in achieving these high standards constituted failure, even though he did not reach this same conclusion in other areas of his life.

These ridiculously high standards represent the dream of all dieters and binge eaters but they simply are not attainable. You can control your eating and your weight but you will never be perfect in this regard. The more you try to be perfect, the less likely you will achieve success.

This may not sound sensible to you but *success means lowering your standards.*

....

HOW BINGE EATING AND SELF-TALK ARE CONNECTED

Talking to yourself in a negative and perfectionistic way leads to negative feelings about yourself, lowered self-esteem, and binge eating. Thoughts, feelings, and behavior are interconnected, but thoughts are the driving force behind both emotional distress and out-of-control eating. This is important to understand because if you change the way you think about food, eating, and your feelings about dieting and weight, you will change your binge-eating patterns.

When you binge and subsequently feel depressed, guilty, anxious, and worthless, your thoughts are dominated by negativity. Because of your negative thoughts, you come to believe that you have no control over your eating and that things are as bad as you imagine them to be. This belief leads to more eating and a continuation of the binge-eating cycle. Because of your perfectionism and low self-esteem, your negative thoughts contain distortions of rational thought that are wrong. Rather than challenge your negative thoughts, you have learned to accept them as fact.

It's as if your worst enemy resided in your mind and was feeding you all kinds of distorted information and lies. You believe these lies and allow them to influence your feelings and your actions. This enemy is telling you that you have no power over food, that you will never succeed, that nothing less than total self-control is necessary for weight control as well as your worth as a person, and that you are addicted to food and will never control your eating. Would you ever say these things to someone? Of course not. You would consider this a cruel form of brainwashing, which it is.

Both the bad part and the good part of this situation is that the enemy from within is you. In other words, to quote the Pogo cartoon-strip character, "We have met the enemy and he is us." Since you are the enemy, you can decide to change this mental monologue to a dialogue. We can put another voice into your mind, one that at least begins to question all of this negativity.

This may be unnatural to you at first but you will be able to do it. Thinking habits are similar to behavioral habits. We can change them both. You think the way you do because that is the way you've always thought. This is not an inborn way of thinking. You learned to think in perfectionistic, all-or-nothing, negative ways and you can unlearn these patterns as well. I see people every day who have successfully changed the way they think about food and eating, and who are now free of the bingeing that kept them prisoners to their overweight and their despair.

....

MINDFUL THINKING AWARENESS— THE FIRST STEP

The first step in changing thought patterns is to increase your awareness of exactly what you are saying to yourself about your eating and your weight. Prior to, during, and after binge eating your mind is very busy with all kinds of thoughts—mostly negative ones. These thoughts are having a very bad influence on your mood and confidence. At the time, you probably have very little awareness of what thoughts are in your head. This is partly due to the mindlessness and "spaced-out" experience that occurs around the time of binge eating.

Your first goal, then, is to increase your awareness of what you are saying to yourself. This can best be accomplished using an ABC approach to analyzing your thoughts regarding food. There are often three elements to circumstances surrounding binge eating. These three ABCs are:

A	**B**	**C**
ADVERSITY	BELIEF	CONSEQUENCE

The **Adversity** refers to the events or circumstances that were occurring at the time. It pertains to what was happening at the time that triggered your food cravings. It could have been that you were alone and your favorite food was available. Perhaps you just had a disagreement with your spouse or children. Maybe you were attending a holiday celebration.

The **Belief** refers to what you are saying to yourself about the events and circumstances. These are your thoughts, attitudes, and perceptions. Let's suppose you were upset about a critical remark your spouse made about your weight. Your thoughts might include, "He makes me so mad. He's always putting me down. He doesn't understand how difficult it is for me to lose weight. What's the use? I'll never be able to please him anyway. I might as well just go ahead and eat." These thoughts are the most important part of your analysis. They are responsible for how you feel and what you do next.

The **Consequence** refers to how you feel and what you do. You might feel upset and depressed and eat a package of cookies.

When analyzing your binge eating in this way, it is important to stop everything you are doing and go off by yourself. Sit quietly, close your eyes, and, as I have advised in earlier chapters, adopt a mindful attitude. Paying attention, being aware, and becoming an observer will all help you discover the details of your craving and binge experience. Your thoughts will only become clear to you if you pay close attention to them through mindfulness. Do not allow any distractions while you are analyzing your mind in this way.

When you are finished, write your discoveries on a piece of paper in the form of the A, B, and C's. Divide the paper into three columns and write the events that happened, your thoughts about those events, and what you felt and what you did.

At first, when binge-eating episodes occur, you should analyze your thoughts by breaking down what happened into these three elements. As you gain more control, analyze your thoughts as they are happening so you can prevent the binge from occurring.

Let's suppose you are 35 pounds overweight and decide to join a health club as part of your weight-control program. You believe that a regularly scheduled aerobics class three times a week will help structure your exercise program and keep you motivated. Since the club is located close to where you live, you'll be able to use the treadmills two other days a week. You walk in with the intention of signing up for a year's membership. Once inside, you notice that almost everyone who is attending the classes and working out is trim and fit. All of a sudden, you feel extremely self-conscious and embarrassed. You feel like hiding under a rock. There are mirrors on the walls and everywhere you look you are conscious of how overweight you are. You panic and leave without signing up. You feel so upset and dejected that on the way home you go to McDonald's and order a bacon cheeseburger, large fries, and a chocolate milkshake.

Let's analyze this situation, using the ABC approach.

A	B	C
Walking into the health club and seeing trim bodies	"Those people must think I look like a blimp. I don't belong here. I'll never look like that. What's the use? I'll never be able to lose weight."	Depressed. Feeling worthless, ate "fast food" and went off my diet.

Your first instinct may be to believe that A caused C. You might think that your experience at the health club caused you to feel depressed and to overeat. This is totally wrong. In reality, B caused C. B *always* causes C. It is your interpretation of the events at the health club, what you were saying to yourself about what happened at the health club, that caused the binge. This is very, very important.

It is unfortunate that you cannot control life's events. However, you can control your thoughts and beliefs about life's events. If you change your thoughts, you can change the way you feel about and react to everything that happens to you. You can control and put a stop to your binge eating and, more specifically, you can control your life.

....

HOW TO CHANGE THE WAY
YOU TALK TO YOURSELF

Once you complete the ABC analysis of your eating, you are ready to change the script of your self-talk. Focus on the B column of your analysis. Take each thought, one at a time. Your goal is to look for negative, distorted thoughts and to challenge them. Your goal is to write a new set of thoughts, a new script. Pretend you are someone else, perhaps your own best friend, when you are doing this.

Let's suppose, while dieting, you ate a bowl of ice cream. The consequence is that you feel guilty and discouraged and then eat the rest of the carton of ice cream. Your thoughts after the first bowl were, "Here I go again. Now I've really blown my diet. What is wrong with me? I'm so stupid. I don't have any willpower and never will."

You must write these thoughts out and then challenge them. You should not allow yourself to get away with this type of thinking. I want you to argue with yourself. You can challenge these irrational, negative thoughts by asking the following questions.

1. What is the evidence for this?

Take the statement, "I've really blown my diet," and look at the facts behind it. As you think about it, realize that one bowl of ice cream (let's suppose you had a cup, which is about two servings) is approxi-

190

mately 300 calories. One instance of eating 300 calories is not "blowing" a diet. In fact, you would have had to eat more than 3,500 calories of ice cream above your dietary level of calories to gain even one pound! Three hundred calories over the long run means nothing. And what about the times you were tempted to eat ice cream and you didn't? Give yourself credit. Change this thought to, "I ate only two servings of ice cream. I did not 'blow' my diet. I am not off my diet. I'm being much too hard on myself."

2. *What are other possible ways to explain what happened?*

Take the statement, "I don't have any willpower." You are assuming that you ate the ice cream because you have a personal deficiency, a character flaw. You are also overgeneralizing. That is, you are assuming that one episode of loss of control means that you never have control. This is simply not the case with you or anyone else. No one is perfect. People who are successful fail from time to time. People who have willpower do not always demonstrate that willpower. Maybe you ate the ice cream because you were stressed out or tired or hungry or simply because you like the taste of ice cream. These are not excuses, these are the facts. It's okay to be overwhelmed by stress or cravings from time to time. This is natural. It happens to everyone. Some people eat under these conditions, some lose their tempers, others drink too much, while some go on shopping sprees and spend too much money.

3. *What are the implications of what I am saying to myself?*

What does "blowing your diet" mean? What does it imply about you? Your thoughts were: "What is wrong with me? I am so stupid. I don't have any willpower and never will." Does eating ice cream really make you stupid? Does it mean you have been transformed into a weak-willed person forever? Of course not. But this is exactly what you are telling yourself. This is your belief at the time. If this belief goes unchallenged, you will assume that you are stupid and weak-willed and act accordingly. You will give up on your diet and yourself. This false belief will continue to influence your actions and your mood.

4. *Are these thoughts doing me any good?*

Even if you believe these thoughts and think they are true, are they doing you any good? Are they helping or hurting you? These are extremely harmful thoughts that are shattering your self-esteem and self-confidence. Remember, these negative thoughts are a prime cause of your binge eating. You must rid yourself of their influence. All you have to do is challenge them, argue with them, and give them up. One way to give them up is to use the mindfulness strategy of "letting go" that I described in Chapter 13.

....

THE CASE OF MELISSA

When I first saw Melissa she was a 24-year-old single woman living in the same small town in eastern North Carolina in which she had grown up. She was living with her parents and working in the account-ing department of a large boat-building company in a nearby city. Melissa was a shy, introverted young woman who had a great deal of weight to lose. At 5 feet 4 inches, her weight of 214 pounds made life un-comfortable.

Physically, she had little energy or stamina. Even mild physical exertion caused shortness of breath. She could only walk short distances. Finding cloth-ing that fit was a major chore. Her weight caused her to be very self-conscious and she rarely socialized.

Melissa had a major binge-eating problem. Binges were often triggered by negative, perfectionistic thinking. In addition, her mother, who had always been thin, was very critical of Melissa's weight and appearance. Melissa binged just about every day. She loved sweets and chocolate in any form.

She had tried diet after diet but had given up two years ago. During that time, her binge eating wors-ened and her weight increased to her present weight of 214 pounds. She only agreed to try again when her physician diagnosed her with borderline diabetes and high blood pressure. Diabetes ran in her family and she wanted to avoid daily insulin injections.

Fortunately, Melissa did not simply try another

standard weight-loss diet. She recognized that she would not be able to lose weight unless she did something about her binge eating. Because of her past dietary failures, she began my program with apprehension but a great deal of determination. We focused mainly on changing her negative thinking since this was a major factor in her binge eating.

Her negative, all-or-nothing thoughts were so ingrained in her mind that they seemed to arise by reflex. If she deviated even a little from her dietary goals, discouraging thoughts would throw her completely off her program for days. Once, she had a craving for chocolate, and even though she did not eat it, she convinced herself that she was weak-willed for even experiencing the craving in the first place.

Melissa did not realize how much influence her thoughts had on her binge eating. In questioning her, I discovered that she had very little awareness of her thoughts. When she binged and I asked her to tell me what she was saying to herself at the time, she had no clue. "I wasn't thinking of anything," she would reply. Once she learned mindfulness and began to pay attention to her thoughts, she learned that there were many, many thoughts in her mind. "I'm amazed to find out there is a continual monologue of thoughts going on in my head and I wasn't even aware of it. When I listen to the negative things I say to myself, I think, 'No wonder you feel so down on yourself and no wonder you eat so much.' "

Melissa began to be more mindful about her thoughts and wrote them down, as instructed. She learned to challenge and argue with these thoughts. She actually enjoyed this process immensely. She envisioned that the voice producing these thoughts was an enemy from within. She saw this enemy as the "old Melissa." The "new Melissa" enjoyed arguing a more positive case and winning.

Here's an example of how Melissa analyzed her thoughts after a binge episode during which she ate three candy bars. Normally, this would have triggered more eating. However, in this case, she was able to be aware of her negative thoughts and successfully rewrite her internal script.

Negative Thought #1

"When it comes to food, I can't control myself."

Better Thought #1

"I control my appetite most of the time. I only lose control every once in a while. I am not perfect and neither is anyone else."

Negative Thought #2

"I have no willpower. I am a weak person."

Better Thought #2

"This is not true. Willpower is not something you have or you don't have. Just because I ate the candy doesn't mean that I'm weak. I am basically a strong person, but not all of the time."

Negative Thought #3

"I'll probably pig out all weekend."

Better Thought #3

"What am I, a fortune-teller? I can get back in control right now. In fact, by writing these new thoughts, I'm feeling better already."

As you can see, Melissa became very adept at challenging her negative thoughts. This new-found power over her mind stimulated a confidence in Melissa that she had not known before. Although she put my entire program into practice, it was mindful mind control that helped her the most. Melissa took control of her binge eating as well as her life. Within the first few weeks of treatment, her binge eating ceased. She began losing weight and continued to lose. Over the next year she did experience three short episodes of binge eating but was able to nip them in the bud using mindful mind control. She now weighs 130 pounds—a weight loss of 84 pounds!

The "new Melissa" truly won the battle against her binge eating and her weight. She is currently married, living in Tampa, and working with her husband in a private accounting firm.

As you have seen in this chapter, mindful mind control is primarily used for breaking negative thoughts that trigger binges or that make you feel so guilty after a binge that they throw you into a relapse. In the next two chapters, I'll show you how to use mindfulness to improve your body image and self-esteem, two important issues in conquering your binge-eating pattern.

CHAPTER 15

....

Body Mindfulness: Discovering a New Body Image

A negative body image and poor self-esteem are major obstacles to your conquering your binge-eating problem. You must improve how you feel about yourself and your body if you are going to defeat your impulses to overeat. In fact, studies show that binge eaters who do not change their extreme concern about weight and shape are unlikely to change.

How important is your body size to you? Let's suppose that you have had several telephone or e-mail conversations with someone but neither of you had met one another. What response would you have if that person said to you, "Tell me about yourself." What would you say? Would your body size be included in your description? Would it be the first thing that comes to your mind? Would your description be positive or negative? Would you list your positive attributes or your shortcomings? If you did mention your body size, would you be embarrassed? Would you be making self-derogatory remarks?

I will show you how to develop a *mindful self-image*, one in which you will look at yourself with a more positive attitude. If you are to succeed at stopping your bingeing, you must expand your definition of self-worth beyond your body size and shape.

....

WHY YOUR BODY IMAGE
MUST IMPROVE

In earlier chapters I discussed how attitudes toward body size in families as well as in society at large contribute to binge-eating disorder. Your battle with food has a great deal to do with your image of yourself. Somewhere along the line you learned to define yourself as a person by your body size and shape. You learned to believe that fat is bad and thin is good. Fat is ugliness and grief while thin is beauty and happiness.

When I ask my clients, "Do you really believe that thin people are happier than overweight people?" they often answer in the affirmative. They truly believe that people who are thin have fewer problems and are generally more content with life, *because they are thin*. Many of my clients feel that happiness, success, and peace of mind are more a matter of body size than attitude, belief in yourself, hard work, competence, relationships with others, or life skills.

Intense dislike and preoccupation with your body size or shape leads to a preoccupation with dieting and with food. You must lose weight not merely to improve health or appearance but to be acceptable to yourself and others. To lose weight means to be worthy. To lose weight means that you are a worthwhile, appreciated person. Weight loss is the only road to happiness and fulfillment. No wonder you become obsessed with dieting and with food.

Once this happens you pave the way for the all-or-nothing pattern of food avoidance versus binge eating. You are either dieting and depriving yourself or going to the other extreme and binge eating. Since body size is so important to your self-worth, negative thoughts about your body send you into a self-destructive pattern of bingeing. A glance in a mirror that results in a barrage of self-critical analysis leads to self-hatred, self-blame, and feelings of defeat. This negativity triggers a binge, which in turn triggers more negativity. Weight gain from the binge reinforces the idea that you are even heavier and more unworthy. By then, you completely give up.

CHANGING THE WAY YOU THINK ABOUT YOUR BODY

Learning to accept who and what you are is an important part of enhancing your feelings of self-worth. You may say, "But how can I learn to accept my body, especially these big hips of mine, when I despise the way I look?" I understand how you feel. I am asking you to accept your body for what it is. You don't have to like the way you look and, indeed, you might want to change the way you look. If your body is larger than you would wish it to be, let's accept that fact and try to do something about it.

If you are like most binge eaters, you judge yourself by the way your body looks. The way we look in a physical sense is certainly part of us and thus part of our image of who we are. But, we are also many other things such as our character, our values, and who we are in relationship to our families, work, and the world in general. But for many reasons, you have come to judge yourself mostly by your body size and shape.

Your overvaluation of your body's appearance may be due to the fact that you have always been overweight. Children and adolescents are very sensitive about themselves, and young egos can be very fragile. Your sensitivity about your body may also be due to what you heard from others as you were growing up. Perhaps others judged and accepted you mostly by your appearance.

Because of your all-or-nothing thinking style, you relate to your weight in one of two opposing ways—total avoidance or obsessive worry and self-contempt. If you don't like your weight or if it disgusts and depresses you, you can deal with it through avoidance. In a childish way, if we don't think about our problems we think they'll go away. You try to deny your weight problem if you answer "yes" to the following questions.

- Do you avoid thinking about or looking at your body?
- Do you avoid weighing yourself?
- Do you avoid looking at yourself in mirrors?
- Do you run in the other direction when someone is taking photographs?
- Are you self-conscious and embarrassed about your body?
- Do you hide your body?
- Do you avoid social or recreational activities because of your weight?

Jan, a 41-year-old client of mine, practiced body avoidance so much so that she eventually began to distort reality. She had always been overweight, but over the past two years her weight ballooned to 245 pounds. Her binge eating was totally out of control. She was so despondent about her weight that she gave up all efforts at dieting. She felt overwhelmed and defeated.

At this point, Jan stopped weighing herself. Getting on the scale had become so traumatic she decided she'd had enough. She didn't want to think about or talk about her weight. Her sister was very concerned about her but whenever she brought up the subject of dieting or weight, Jan refused to talk about it. She wanted to be left alone.

Her denial became extreme. One day as she looked at a recent family photograph taken on Thanksgiving day, she remarked with all sincerity, "Oh my goodness, it looks like I've put on a few pounds." Jan was actually over 100 pounds over-weight at the time.

While avoidance and denial is not the answer to a better body image, neither is obsessive worrying. Overconcern and oversensitivity to your body can limit your life in many ways. You may relate every-thing to your body shape and size. Every social event becomes a nightmare. Buying a new outfit for a spe-cial occasion becomes a dreadful experience. You never would think of putting on a bathing suit. I have had married women clients who, for years, have undressed in the dark so their husbands would not see their naked bodies.

ACCEPTANCE: THE FIRST STEP TOWARD CHANGE

Acceptance of who and what you are is the first step in changing your body image and eventually in over-coming your binge-eating disorder. To accept your-self for who you are both physically and mentally, you must confront your weight. You must stop deny-ing and come face-to-face with your weight. I know this might be very difficult for you but it is essential if you are to move forward and to change. Change is difficult and often painful but you'll emerge on the other side of that pain as a stronger person.

Your first impulse will be to avoid confrontation. I have had clients say to me, "Why should I think about and look at my body? It depresses me. I'm grotesque. I hate my body." The important thing for you to remember is that *to accept your body in a non-judgmental, mindful way does not mean that you have to like your body.* You must accept yourself as you are. If you binge eat and are 50 pounds overweight, that is the way things are.

I am not trying to depress you or make you feel bad about yourself. I am asking you to accept yourself. You don't have to like or love yourself. You can say, "I accept the fact that I am very overweight. I don't want to be overweight, and I don't like the fact that I am this way. But I accept it." Once you accept this fact on an emotional level, you will be ready to change. Self-contempt and self-hatred about your body simply make you feel worse. It's time to let go of this self-punishment.

Most people assume that they cannot accept themselves until they lose weight. It is true that people who learn to control their binge eating and lose weight learn to think more positively about themselves. This will happen to you as well. However, you must start the process before weight loss occurs. In fact, you must start accepting yourself first, before changes occur. Otherwise, changes in binge eating and weight loss may never happen.

Here's how to begin, how to put mindfulness into practice to increase your self-esteem and improve your body image.

....

THE BODY SCAN: ACHIEVING A NEW BODY IMAGE

Mindfulness can be applied to your body image through a technique known as the **Body Scan**. Mentally scanning your body in a mindful, nonjudgmental way allows you to begin the process of acceptance that I've been talking about.

The Body Scan is simply looking at and thinking about your body in a mindful way. Remember, mindfulness involves paying attention, increasing awareness, focusing on the moment, and adopting an observational, nonjudgmental attitude. I will be asking you to pay attention to your body in this way.

To practice the Body Scan, choose a time when you are by yourself and you will not be disturbed for at least 20 to 30 minutes. Lie down in bed, on a sofa, or in a reclining chair. Choose a time when you are not sleepy because it is important to stay alert during this exercise. Clear your mind, close your eyes, and relax. Take a few slow, deep breaths.

Begin to scan your body in a slow, progressive fashion. Begin with your fingers. Focus your attention on your fingers using a mindful attitude. Pay attention to them. Be aware of them. Focus on what they feel like at this moment in time. Remember to remain an observer, not a judge. Pay attention to whatever physical sensations, emotions, or thoughts you are experiencing as you focus on your fingers.

205

Now move your attention to your hands. Stay there for a few moments and then move to your wrists, then your forearms, then your upper arms, then your shoulders. Spend a few minutes focusing on each body part in a nonjudgmental, mindful way. Be aware of the specific details of your experiences with each body part. Stay observational, but be aware of thoughts associated with various body parts.

For example, let's suppose that when focusing on your upper arms, you think, "My arms are so flabby and unattractive. I wish I could wear sleeveless dresses but I know I look horrible in them." Be aware of that thought but do not become caught up in it. Do not let that thought carry you away. Instead, take the attitude of an observer who might say, "It's interesting that I would have such a thought about my arms." Your arms, even if they are flabby, are your arms. They are neither positive nor negative. They just are!

Continue moving through your body, focusing on these body parts in the following sequence:

neck
chin
jaws
mouth/lips
nose
cheeks
ears
eyes
forehead

head
upper back
lower back
sides
chest / breasts
stomach/waist
genitals
hips
buttocks
thighs
knees
calves
ankles
feet
toes

As your mind goes from one body part to another, imagine that your breathing is moving through your entire body.

After you have finished, spend another few moments focusing on your entire body. Accept what you are experiencing, don't judge. Don't label. Pretend you are an objective, open-minded scientist observing a human body for the first time. Your viewpoint should be one of curiosity, not judgment.

Focus on your breathing. Breathe in a slow, steady, relaxed manner. Imagine that as you inhale you are breathing in positive energy that gives your body, mind, and spirit a feeling of strength and vitality. When you exhale, imagine that negative thoughts and feelings are leaving your body.

Do not allow your mind to wander. Stay with your body and your breathing. If distracting thoughts occur, notice what they are but let them go. If your thought is, "I shouldn't be lying here like this. I have a million things to do this afternoon," pay attention to that thought but let it go away. Don't get caught up in it. Don't let it control your mind. You can think about these matters when you are finished. Concentrated focus is a key to the Body Scan.

When you first practice this exercise you may find your mind focusing on the negative. In spite of your best efforts you may have self-critical thoughts about your body. When you think about your thighs or buttocks you may begin to feel tense. Your thoughts may be, "My thighs are huge. I'll never look normal. I'll never be able to lose weight." In fact, these negative thoughts about your body may have, in the past, served as emotional triggers for binge eating. This is why it is so essential to become more aware of this negative thinking and to change it.

If you are aware of negative body thoughts during the Body Scan, don't worry. You are not in the habit of thinking about your body in an accepting, mindful way. Your typical thoughts about your body are critical and negative. That is what is familiar to you.

Because of your negative self-image, you are accustomed to convincing yourself that you are unworthy of respect. In fact, positive thoughts about your body may scare you. You may even react to compliments from others in a negative way.

The secret to the effectiveness of the Body Scan is

repetition. You cannot expect to practice this exercise once or twice and feel more positively about your body. In fact, after the first time you do it, you may feel a little tense and uneasy. This is especially true if you have been avoiding your body or denying your shape or weight.

Success comes through many, many repetitions. You must stick with it. Practice as often as you can and gradually you will begin to experience a change in how you feel about your body. You will begin to accept your body as it really is. At this point, you will be able to set about the changes that are needed to change your life.

Remember, acceptance of your body does not mean that you have given up your battle with weight loss. Rather, it indicates that you are stronger than ever to fight that battle. It's okay to be concerned about your weight, but I don't want you to be obsessed with it.

....

CONFRONTING YOUR
MIRROR IMAGE

Another technique that can help you deal with your body more directly is the **Mirror Image Technique**. First, with your clothes on, stand in front of a full-length mirror. Take a slow, deep breath. Stay calm. If you have been avoiding mirrors, you might feel a little anxious. This is perfectly normal. Your anxiety will gradually fade away. Clear your thoughts and adopt an observational, mindful attitude. Take another slow, deep breath and relax your body.

Take a long, slow look at yourself. Start with your feet and gradually work your way up your body. As you go from your feet to your ankles to your calves to your knees and so on, look at each part of your body. Pay attention to it and be aware of it. What does each part of your body look like? As you look at and think about each part of your body, how do you feel? Most important, what are you saying to yourself? Are you judging? Are you being critical?

Make sure you pay attention to positive self-evaluations. Which aspects of your body are you satisfied with? Which parts are you proud of?

Be aware of your self-talk during this exercise. It often helps to write your thoughts on paper as you are looking at your reflection. List the three parts of your body that you like the most and what thoughts you have about these parts. Now, do the same thing for the three parts of your body that you like the least.

When you are finished, look carefully at what you have written. First, focus on your list of positive qualities. Binge eaters usually are so negative about their bodies that they disregard positive attributes. You might be proud of the texture or color of your hair, or the smoothness or your skin, or the gracefulness of your hands. Because you avoid thinking about your body or you focus so much on the body parts that you dislike, you ignore the physical aspects that you admire. Be specific about what you are saying to yourself about these positives. Be careful not to discount positive self-talk with such remarks as, "Sure my eyes are attractive, but my waist is huge."

Next, review what you have written about the three body areas you dislike the most. Remember, it's okay to say, "I don't like my big hips. I wish they were smaller." It's not okay to say, "I despise my hips. I look like a freak. I wish I could look like that model I saw on television last night." Hating your hips only makes you feel worse about yourself. Saying that you look like a freak only serves to make you feel different. Dreaming of looking like a model who is genetically programmed to have small, boyish hips will only depress and disappoint you because it is unrealistic.

The most important fact for you to remember is that *you do not feel frustrated and depressed because of your hips, you feel frustrated and depressed by what you are telling yourself about your hips.* If you change your self-talk, you will begin to change how you feel about your body and eventually yourself.

It is not necessary to become Pollyannish about the matter, convincing yourself that you love your body. The important point is that you need to become more realistic and accepting. You must start to have a different conversation with yourself. You must begin to put another voice in your head that says something such as, "What are you doing to yourself? Is all this self-hatred doing you any good? Even if you don't like your body, is reminding yourself of this fact every day helping or hurting you?"

211

....

EXERCISE AND BODY IMAGE

In Chapter 17 I will outline my mindful exercise plan for you. Exercise puts you in touch with all aspects of your body in such a way that you will become more aware and accepting of your physical being. Studies have shown that people who exercise regularly (not strenuously) have a greater appreciation of their bodies. Exercise will not only help you lose weight but will also help to change your body shape. With time, you will be more aware of the look and feel of your body and appreciate the changes that will occur. You will also become more accepting of which body dimensions you can change and which you cannot.

CHAPTER 16

The Mindful Self: Improving Your Self-Esteem

Self-esteem refers to your sense of worth or value as a person. It is composed of two basic elements: (1) how much you believe in yourself, and (2) how much you respect yourself. Let's look at each element to find out how you can believe in and respect yourself to a greater degree.

HOW MUCH YOU BELIEVE IN YOURSELF

Belief in your competence as an individual is very important in determining not only how you feel about yourself but also how you cope with challenges in your life. In the field of psychology we use the term *self-efficacy belief* to refer to the confidence you have in your ability to successfully master specific challenges in your life. What we find is that people do not

213

exhibit an overall sense of confidence in all areas of their lives. Rather, self-efficacy beliefs tend to be specific to specific situations. You may believe strongly in yourself in certain areas of your life but have very little confidence or self-esteem in other areas.

To illustrate this point, I'll tell you about a study I conducted with colleagues at the University of South Carolina. We were trying to find out what differences existed in self-efficacy beliefs between overweight binge eaters and those who were overweight but did not binge eat. Out of a group of overweight men and women whose average age was 49 years, 36 percent experienced significant binge-eating problems. We administered a test called the Weight Efficacy Lifestyle Questionnaire, designed to measure the confidence an individual has in successfully dealing with a variety of eating situations. For example, the test asks individuals to rate their level of confidence in refraining from eating tempting foods when they are angry, when they are celebrating, when they are alone, when there is social pressure to eat, when a lot of food is available, etc.

The overall scores showed that the binge eaters had much lower confidence in their ability to control their eating than the overweight nonbinge eaters. The binge eaters rated themselves the lowest on their ability to resist eating in circumstances involving emotional distress such as anger, tension, and depression, as well as situations involving physical discomfort such as fatigue or pain. The binge eaters had more confidence in their willpower when they were in social situations in which tempting food was available.

We also found gender differences in these self-efficacy ratings. In particular, women felt much less confident than men in resisting food when they were emotionally upset. In other studies we have also found that women experience much more guilt and frustration *after* a binge than do men. Compared to men, women's binge eating seems to be much more tied into emotions in general and self-esteem and body image in particular. Society's standards allow men more latitude regarding their weight and eating behavior than women. A moderately overweight man who is eating a great deal might be considered to have a "hearty appetite" whereas a woman in similar circumstances might be viewed with disdain.

Just like the people in my study, you may find that your confidence in controlling your eating varies depending on what situations we are talking about. You expect to succeed in some situations but not in others. Most people accept this fact and take it for granted. If you lack self-esteem, rather than see a balance of your abilities and shortcomings, you allow your weaknesses to rule your image of yourself. Even if you were to have a positive thought about self-efficacy in one area of your life, you would quickly discount that ability by thinking of an area in which you think you are deficient.

Let's suppose you think, "I bet I could handle that assignment at work as well as Joan. In fact, I know I could. I am a better organizer and problem solver than she is." Your poor image of yourself might lead you to answer with, "So what? She's as thin as a rail and always eats salad for lunch while I'm pigging out on baby-back ribs. I have no control over myself when it comes to food, and I'm as heavy as a horse. I'm no good at anything."

Just as I mentioned in Chapter 14, you must not overgeneralize. You must separate your strong and weak areas and not let the weak ones cancel out what you are good at. Remind yourself that everyone experiences a balance between what they feel competent in doing and what they do not. People with low self-esteem allow the negatives to overshadow the positives. Don't allow this to happen.

Belief in yourself is important for two basic reasons. First, people who believe in their competence have greater self-esteem. Since this is the case, you can improve your self-esteem by learning to believe in your capabilities. If you improve your self-esteem, you greatly improve your chances of overcoming your binge-eating disorder. Second, under conditions of adversity, people who have more confidence in their abilities try harder to overcome that hardship. If your expectation is that you will not be able to overcome a difficult situation or temptation, you will give up quickly without a struggle.

This is why belief is so important as far as binge eating is concerned. If you learn my mindful-eating techniques but fail to apply them, you will never be able to succeed. You will have given up before you begin. Unfortunately, this is exactly what you've experienced in the past. We must put those days behind you once and for all.

I realize that you may be thinking that the reason you lack confidence in your ability to resist binge eating in high-risk situations is that you have failed to do so in the past. Your present belief is weak because you have learned from experience that you will binge, especially when you are upset, tired, lonely, or bored. You must close the door to the past. What has happened in the past does not matter. Because of your low self-esteem your memory will only high-light your failures from the past. Just as I pointed out in Chapter 10 on mindful willpower, you have had many episodes of successful self-control, but you haven't given yourself credit for them. Your mental picture of your level of success and competence is just plain wrong and distorted. You have been trying to prove to yourself how unsuccessful you are most of your life. This is why your self-esteem is so low.

The "new" you is not going to do that anymore. You are going to regularly take stock of your strengths. You are going to be more mindful of the times in which you are competent and successful either with food or with anything else in your life. As we discussed in Chapter 14 on mindful mind control, you are going to challenge your negative thoughts about yourself and not let yourself get away with your continual put-downs. You deserve better than that, especially from yourself. The concept of "de-serving better" brings us to the second element of self-esteem, namely, *respect for yourself.*

....

HOW MUCH YOU RESPECT YOURSELF

To feel worthy as a person you must begin to respect yourself. I would bet that when it comes to your conversations with yourself about your personal value, you are your own worst enemy. You would never say what you say to yourself to anyone else. Why? Because you would consider it unfair, unkind, and downright cruel.

To regain respect for yourself, your mission must include: (1) finding your true character, (2) being true to yourself, and (3) taking charge of your life.

FINDING YOUR TRUE CHARACTER

To feel valuable as a person you must know who you are. Do you? Are you mindful of your true character? What makes you unique? What makes you *you*?

Your true self refers to those characteristics about you that are stable and steady. They are there no matter what. They are dimensions of yourself that are part of you regardless of where you happen to be, who you are with, how heavy you are, or how old you are.

It is important to find your true character because it is important for you to define yourself. If you are aware of who and what you are and you accept and acknowledge it, you are defining yourself. If you have a hazy image of yourself, then you allow the world around you to determine who you are. Circumstances, people, and the ups and downs of life determine how you feel about yourself. Under these conditions, your feelings about your self-worth will vary considerably on a day-to-day basis. If you are having a "good" day, if things are going your way, you'll feel worthy. If people are positive and accepting in their interactions with you, you'll feel worthy.

The problem with this state of affairs is probably obvious to you. Life is seldom a bed of roses. In fact, life can be quite difficult. People can be selfish, unkind, manipulative, and deceitful. Circumstances can go against us. Bad things happen to good people and all people for that matter. If you allow the world to define your character, your self-image will be on a roller-coaster ride. You'll be up some days and down others. Your "up" days won't make you feel much better about yourself, because your positive feelings have nothing to do with *you*. They have nothing to do with your efforts, abilities, or character. You are like a feather in the wind, being blown about by life's happenstances.

It is impossible to establish adequate self-esteem under these conditions. Whenever you feel worthwhile, it is because the world says you are, not because you feel you are. And, you must wait for the world to decide when and how long you are worthy.

To establish self-worth, you must look inside yourself. You must look for your inner character, who you are, regardless of the world. This may be a new approach for you. You may avoid looking at *who* you are just as you avoid looking at *what* you are by not acknowledging your body.

Just as you used the Body Scan (described in Chapter 15) to become more mindful of your body image, you can practice the **Self Scan** to become more aware of your character. Schedule about 20 to 30 minutes and sit quietly by yourself. Take a slow, deep breath and close your eyes. Adopt a mindful attitude. Pay attention, be aware, focus on the moment, and become an observer, not a judge. Let go of the past and future. Let go of the outside world. Turn your attention inward. Your goal is to find the true you. Who are you? What is your character? Let the answers come to you. Be patient. You are an observer, looking in at yourself. Be aware of whatever comes into your mind.

For example, you might think, "I am a giving, caring person. I am a creative person. I am often insincere. I am an intelligent person. I am a hard-working person. I always try to do my best in whatever I do. I try to please others. I am sometimes untruthful. I am impatient." You are looking for whatever characteristics come to your mind. You are not judging. You are not separating out the good from the bad, but are observing. The characteristic of "I am often insincere" is as much a part of you as "I am a giving, caring person." I want you to pay attention to your character and accept it.

Just as in the Body Scan, when you accepted your body even though you may not have liked all parts of it, the same is true for the Self Scan. There may be parts of your character you dislike. That's perfectly all right as long as you acknowledge them.

When you are practicing the Self Scan it is important not to judge or disclaim aspects of your character. You are judging if you say, "I am intelligent but certainly not all the time." Just focus on being intelligent. If you were intelligent all of the time you would be an individually unique person. You would be perfect as far as intelligence is concerned. Perfection does not exist. Let's suppose that one morning you told me you were intelligent. That afternoon, you did something very stupid. Would you then return to me and say, "I made a mistake this morning when I told you I was intelligent. I just did a dumb thing so I guess I must not be intelligent anymore"? Of course you wouldn't. You would reason that even the most intelligent person does stupid things from time to time just as the most caring person may occasionally act in a self-centered way.

As a person who has low self-esteem, this distinction may evade you. You probably do tell yourself that one instance of less than perfect actions means that you are imperfect. As a binge eater I know you tell yourself that one instance of overindulgence proves you are devoid of willpower and that you are a failure. During the Self Scan you should be looking for who you are most of the time, not all of the time.

While you are searching for who you are, it is also a good idea to give mindful thought to *who you want to be*. What kind of true character would you like to have? In this way, you can accept who you are, but, at the same time, set your sights on who you want to be.

After 20 or 30 minutes of the Self Scan, open your eyes and write a list of the results of your self-analysis. Use the following categories to guide you:

Who I Am (list all of your personal characteristics):

Who I Want to Be (list all of the personal characteristics you would like to have):

BEING TRUE TO YOURSELF

In order to respect yourself you must be true to yourself. You must present to the world the true, honest, and sincere version of yourself. You must not live your life being a people-pleaser. If you are unable to judge yourself as worthy, then you become desperate to be found worthy by others. You try to please them so you will be accepted and liked. You avoid conflict at all costs. You live the life you think others expect you to live.

Elizabeth had spent her life pleasing others. She and her husband had children early in their marriage, and by the time she was 50, Elizabeth's children were grown and married with children of their own. Her husband had built a successful computer software business over the years. His dream was to sell his company in a year, retire at an early age, buy a yacht, and travel the world.

Elizabeth came to me for help because on her fiftieth birthday she had decided that she was ready for a change. She was not happy with her life. She had always been 15 to 20 pounds overweight but over the last two years had put on another 20 pounds. At 5 feet 6 inches tall and weighing 178 pounds, she felt like a frump. She tried to diet but could not sustain her motivation. She would diet for a day or two and then binge on ice cream or candy. The first thing she said to me was, "You've got to help me. My eating is out of control and so is my life. I even keep my binge eating a secret from my husband and children. I feel so guilty."

Elizabeth had been the oldest of three children. She had grown up as "the good girl," always doing the right thing, always trying to please her parents. Her parents were very meticulous people who expected their children to be near perfect. Even though Elizabeth rarely misbehaved, always brought home good grades, continually helped out around the house, and cared for her younger brother and sister, her mother was very critical of her. Being a perfectionist, her mother was quick to find fault with Elizabeth. If she cleaned up the kitchen, her mother could always find something that wasn't quite clean enough. Her mother was not mean-spirited, she simply believed that too much praise would spoil her children.

Even as an adult, Elizabeth tried to please everyone. She was the perfect mother and wife. She always put her own needs last in order to do for the family. She was the first to help friends in need even if it meant that she was inconvenienced. Now that her parents were getting older, she was the one who cared for them, even though her brother and sister lived closer to them. By age 50 she had realized that the more she did for others the more that was expected of her. People took it for granted that she would help and would frequently take advantage of her good nature. She was beginning to feel used and abused but could not get herself to do anything about it. It was at times like this, when she felt that life was unfair to her, that she would binge.

She felt she had no life of her own. She had always done what others wanted her to do. She rarely disagreed with anyone, even when she had a strong difference of opinion. She allowed her husband to take the lead in most family decisions. Of late, his retirement plans were causing her anxiety. She loved spending time with her grandchildren, and the idea of extended world travel did not appeal to her. Her husband's greatest love was boating and he had plans for them to spend most of their spare time on the yacht he was going to buy. Elizabeth had never enjoyed the water but had never told her husband. The future looked bleak to her. She felt trapped. On top of everything else, her weight problem was getting worse by the week.

Self-esteem was a major focus of my binge-eating treatment plan for Elizabeth. This was because Elizabeth was leading a false life. She was leading a lie. She needed to find out who she was and what kind of person she wanted to be. I helped her discover her true self and encouraged her to decide what type of life she wanted to live.

However, thinking about yourself and what you really want out of life is not enough. The important step is to put your desires into action. It was at this point that Elizabeth became panicky. She wanted to be more direct and sincere with others but she was afraid. I convinced her that to be true to herself she was going to have to behave in ways that demonstrated this trait. This is extremely important. When you act in ways that show you respect yourself and are true to yourself, you will gain self-esteem. Changes in your thoughts and behavior come first and self-esteem follows.

The important question for Elizabeth was, "What will I have to *do* to be true to myself, my feelings, and my needs? What specific actions are necessary?" These were some of her answers.

I must say "no" more often to those who are taking advantage of my kindness

I must express my thoughts directly when I disagree with someone

I must tell my brother and sister that they must provide more help with our parents

I must tell my husband that I do not want to travel as much as he does

If people make me angry or hurt my feelings I must tell them how I feel

I must tell my husband and children about my binge eating and not keep it a secret

I must stick up for myself and talk about what I want and need

At first, Elizabeth was hesitant about these changes. "What will people think of me?" she asked. She worried that others would think she was selfish. "What if they don't like the real me? What if they get mad? What if they reject me?" she wondered. We discussed her fears and I convinced her that most of her concerns were unfounded and would not occur. However, I warned her that when she began to be true to herself, some people may not like it. Some may think she is selfish and may not like her. It may take her husband time to adjust to a more direct, honest, and assertive wife. This is all part of life. With time, however, she will learn to respect herself and, in turn, others will gain respect for her also.

This is exactly what happened. Little by little, Elizabeth began to act like a more authentic person. She couldn't believe how much it changed her feelings about herself. She began to feel free. She began to feel in control of her life. She felt like a heavy load had been lifted from her shoulders. She even began to have a delightful dream in which she was an eagle, escaping from captivity, flying free high in the sky.

As Elizabeth took control of her life in a more honest, genuine way, her binge eating stopped completely. She lost 35 pounds and had never felt better in her life. She and her husband reached a compromise about yachting as well as traveling. Elizabeth enrolled in a local college and completed her degree in English literature, a dream she had given up on years ago.

Make your own list of "Being True to Yourself" actions and begin to put them into practice. Change is difficult but it will set you free. You deserve to live the life you want to live. Being a more direct, honest, and genuine person—being true to yourself—will enhance your feelings of self-respect and self-worth more than you know. Begin today.

TAKING CHARGE OF YOUR LIFE

The third way to gain respect for yourself is to begin the process of taking charge of your life. Once you decide to be more genuine about your true thoughts and feelings, the notion of taking charge of your life will come naturally to you.

The psychological concept known as *locus of control* is essential to self-esteem. "Locus" refers to "place" or "focal point." Your focal point of control is either *internal* or *external*. To determine whether you are internal or external, you must ask yourself the question, "Who is in charge of my life?" External people think that their lives are mostly controlled by other people, circumstances, or chance events. Internal people believe their lives are controlled primarily by themselves and their own thoughts and actions.

If I asked, "Who's in charge of your health?" and your said, "My doctor is," you would have given me an external answer. An internal answer would be,

"My doctor is my medical advisor and consultant but I am ultimately responsible for my health."

Internal people attribute changes they make in their lives to their own efforts. Externals give the credit to someone or something else. If a friend says, "You've lost weight. You look terrific. How did you do it?" an external person would begin talking about the diet they were following. They would give details about the menu plans and recipes as if they had found a magic pill. The internal person would begin talking about herself. She would say, "I made up my mind to do something about my weight. I bought a book that told me how to do it and I have been making healthier food choices and exercising every day. I feel great."

We know for a fact that improvements in yourself that you attribute to your own efforts are longer lasting than those you attribute to others. As you overcome binge eating you must realize that it is because of your own determination and effort. If this book has helped you, I am pleased. However, it was up to you to purchase this book and to implement the program I have outlined for you. *Binge Buster! Stop Out-of-Control Eating and Lose Weight* served as a tool or a road map. You are going to be successful because of *you*. It is important for you to think this way and even talk about your success in this way.

People who are internal in the way they think and talk about their lives have higher self-esteem than those who are external. To increase self-esteem you must begin to think of yourself as being in charge of your life. More important, you must begin to take charge of your life. You must decide what it is you want, what makes you happy, and then go after it. Externals wait for life to happen to them. Internals make things happen.

Clients often say to me, "But I'll never be able to take charge of my life. I don't have the confidence or self-esteem." I remind them of what I have been telling you all along: behavioral change = self-esteem change. If you change your actions, if you begin to take control of your life, one step at a time, you will increase your self-esteem. If you wait until your self-esteem magically improves for you to begin to act differently, nothing will happen. Remember,

SELF-ESTEEM IS BASED ON HOW YOU THINK AND ACT

You can change the way you think and act. All you have to do is make up your mind.

I want your life to be more fulfilling. I want you to control your own destiny. If your life is in a rut, let's change it. Don't be like the young man who went to a fortune-teller to learn about his future: "You will be poor and unhappy until you are 50 years of age," said the fortune-teller. The dismayed young man asked, "Oh, no. Then what will happen?" The fortune teller replied, "Then, you'll get used to it!" Well, I don't want you to sit back passively and accept whatever life deals you. We're going to change all that.

The key to taking control is **lifestyle balancing**. People with self-esteem have developed a balance in their lives between their "Wants" and their "Shoulds." "Wants" consist of anything you do that brings you pleasure, joy, relaxation, peace, or exhilaration. They are things you do that make you feel good. "Shoulds" are the responsibilities, obligations, and challenges of life.

To feel worthy and content we must achieve an adequate balance between these two areas of our lives. Our lives will feel out of control if we have too many "Shoulds" and few, if any, "Wants." We will feel overwhelmed. Under these conditions, food could take on much more importance than it should. Bingeing on food may become your outlet. It may be the only "Want" you have, so, especially on days when your "Shoulds" pile up even more than usual, you will binge. This is another reason why lifestyle balancing is so important in your battle against binge eating. If we remove binge eating from your "Wants" list, you must have replacements to compensate.

Some people actually have too many "Wants" and not enough "Shoulds." Take the case of someone who is retired. They can do whatever they like. They can spend the day enjoying themselves or doing nothing for that matter. While we all need pleasure and joy in our lives, we also need a sense of obligation and challenge. Challenge drives and motivates us. Obligation to someone or something beyond ourselves gives us purpose and meaning.

Take out a sheet of paper and divide it into two

columns labeled "Wants" and "Shoulds." Under the "Wants" column, list all of the things you do on a day-to-day basis that give you pleasure, joy, excitement, or comfort. For these activities, pleasure should be derived mostly from the process of doing them, not what they accomplish. Some examples would be gardening, reading, eating, listening to music, playing with your children, or browsing through antique shops.

Under the "Shoulds" column, list all of your daily activities that you would consider obligations, responsibilities, or challenges. The emphasis of these activities would primarily be outcome rather than process. These activities are designed to accomplish something for yourself or for others. Even though they are obligations, you might enjoy some of them. However, they are primarily goal-oriented in nature.

Look at your lists and decided which column you need to work on to put your life in better balance. Do you, like most people, have too many obligations and few pleasures? Has food taken on too much importance because of this imbalance? If so, the next step is to brainstorm a list of potential "Wants" to better balance your life.

This exercise is a bit like having a midlife crisis, or any-age crisis for that matter. Every ten years, when we complete another decade in our lives, we spend our birthdays contemplating the meaning of life. We ask, "Where have I been? What is my life all about right now? Where am I going in life?" What I am asking you to do is to look at your "Wants" and

"Shoulds" more often. More important, I want you to do something about any imbalance you find. The "action" part of this plan is important at any age.

My father lived a long, healthy life, living until the age of 94. When he reached 90, we had a big celebration for him. Usually a cheerful, positive person, he seemed depressed that day. I thought perhaps he was despondent about his age, caught up in thoughts about his life being over and death being near. In trying to console him, I learned that he wasn't thinking about death at all. At the ripe old age of 90, he was having a midlife crisis! He was reminiscing about the many years of his life as well as reviewing his current pleasures and challenges. Most important, he was filling in the gaps of his "Wants" and "Shoulds" lists and planning for his future. One of his main goals was to write his memoirs, sharing the history of his life from his birth year of 1900 to the present.

Expand your horizons and dream your dreams. Decide what your "Wants" and "Shoulds" list should look like. If you are looking for pleasures, think about any enjoyable activities that you have done in the past (even as a child). Perhaps there are things you've always wanted to do. Then, begin scheduling time to sample these experiences. If you've always wanted to play a musical instrument or take an art class, look into classes in your community. Put your dreams into action. Much of the joy of "Wants" lies in the anticipation as much as the doing.

Let's look for a moment at what might get in the way of your taking charge of your life. The availability of time might be a realistic consideration. You might be a very busy, involved person who is overwhelmed with responsibilities. Begin by looking at your obligations and consider changing them. Do you need to be responsible for all of them? Can you delegate any? Can you simply stop doing some of them? Are you doing more than your share? Do you need to be more direct and honest and express your own needs to others? Do you need to start saying "no"?

Because of your low self-esteem you may hesitate to live your dreams due to a fear of failure. You may ask, "What if I take art lessons and I'm no good at it?" The answer is simply, "So what?" Begin to live more mindfully. Enjoy the experience of being creative, not the product you are creating. Stop judging yourself. Pay attention, be aware, and simply live.

Begin your journey of believing in yourself and respecting yourself now. Your self-esteem will soar to new heights. Your life will be happier. You'll be in control of your own destiny. You also will not need to binge any longer. Binge eating will be part of the "old" you that doesn't exist anymore.

CHAPTER 17

....

Mindful Exercise

I am sure you know that exercise is a key ingredient in losing weight. Weight loss is very difficult to achieve without it. In fact, consistent exercise is the number one predictor of success in keeping weight off once you lose it.

It is also important for you to understand that daily exercise will help you overcome binge eating. As you will see, you don't need to do very much exercise to help you in this regard. Consistency is the key. So, even if you do not like to exercise, don't worry.

I find that binge eaters fall into two categories. There are those who hate exercise and have always hated it. If you have a lot of weight to lose or if you have been overweight most of your life, exercise may always have been physically difficult for you. If you are 50 pounds overweight and out of shape, exercise is not comfortable at first. Your feet hurt, your knees hurt, and you get out of breath easily. To you, exercise seems like bad-tasting medicine. You know you have to do it, but you dread it. It is especially disconcerting when you realize you will have to exercise for the rest of your life. If you are in this category, I can guarantee that my mindful exercise routine will be different. It is designed to take your mind off the negatives of exercise.

Other binge eaters enjoy exercise. They throw themselves into it with a vengeance. People in this category have a potential problem with exercise because of their all-or-nothing thinking. They either exercise all the time or not at all. They are on-again/off-again exercisers because, if they binge, they become discouraged and stop exercising. If you are in this category, mindful exercise will help you become more moderate and consistent in your approach to physical activity.

Occasionally, binge eaters use excessive exercise to compensate for binge eating. Overeating is followed by long exercise sessions to undo the caloric damage resulting from the binge. This pattern is more typical of bulimia, a more severe eating disorder in which people force themselves to vomit after an episode of overeating. Bulimics also exercise to excess after bingeing.

If you have binge-eating disorder, you are more likely to discontinue exercising after bingeing because of depression and guilt. However, binge eating may occasionally drive you to excessive exercise. I remember a client of mine with this problem who is an attorney in New York City. She felt so despondent after a

Sunday night binge that she cancelled her appoint-
ments Monday morning and walked, nonstop, for
four hours. She was determined to compensate for the
1,000 extra calories she had eaten. She told me, "I had
to make up for what I had done wrong. I not only
wanted to burn the calories but also punish myself for
being so weak." Fortunately, I convinced her that this
perfectionistic, negative thinking was destructive. She
was giving in to her all-or-nothing thinking.

It is certainly all right to exercise moderately after
binge eating. It may help you regain control of yourself. You must avoid extremes of behavior during which
you are exercising way too much or not at all. Getting
into the habit of such severe compensation when you
binge can make your eating problem worse and push
you toward the more serious problem of bulimia.

WHY EXERCISE HELPS
YOU AVOID BINGE EATING

Before I describe mindful exercise, let's examine the
four reasons why exercise can help you defeat your
binge problems.

1. Exercise focuses your attention away from food.

As a veteran dieter, too much of your life has focused
on avoiding food, counting calories, and restraining

your appetite. This is a totally negative approach and, in fact, only part of the solution to weight management. Your weight is a function of the balance between both caloric input and caloric output. Most weight-control experts feel that the output side of the equation is actually more important than the input side.

This is exactly the premise of my best-selling book *The New Hilton Head Metabolism Diet.* Regular moderate physical activity such as walking not only burns calories but also stimulates your metabolism. The form of exercise that I will be recommending burns maximum calories with minimal effort *and* stimulates your resting metabolism. Resting metabolism refers to the number of calories your body burns just to keep you alive. You burn calories even when you are sleeping. But the proper exercise program can help your body burn calories not only while you are exercising but hours later, even when you are sitting or lying down.

Unlike food avoidance, exercise is a positive action. It is something you are doing rather than something you are not doing.

2. Exercise improves your body image.

Moving your body as part of any form of physical activity provides you with more physical energy and stamina. People who exercise on a regular basis begin to feel better about their bodies. As you learned in Chapter 15, improving your body image is an important element in overcoming binge eating.

Exercise also increases your awareness of your body, which is an essential ingredient in your being more accepting of who you are. You can develop a better feeling for your body by using the Body Scan technique (described in Chapter 15) while your body is in motion. Mindful walking allows you to get in touch with the physical side of your being, something you may avoid because of your weight.

3. Exercise reduces stress.

Mindful exercise reduces anxiety and frustration and leads to enhanced feelings of well-being. Exercise is often prescribed as part of the treatment regimen for mild to moderate depression. Since anxiety, frustration, and depression can lead to loss of control over food, anything that helps reduce these feelings will help control binge eating.

One reason why exercise alleviates negative emotions is that regular physical activity changes brain chemistry. Exercise stimulates your brain's production of the hormone norepinephrine. This hormone helps regulate emotional stability. People with balanced emotions have high levels of norepinephrine while chronically depressed people have very low levels.

Regular exercise also stimulates the production of endorphins and serotonin in your body. Endorphins are referred to as "natural opiates" because they are actually morphinelike substances that our brains produce. Endorphins give us a feeling of well-being or a natural high. As you learned in Chapter 6, serotonin is a brain chemical that calms and soothes. You may crave carbohydrates such as cookies, ice cream, and candy because these foods cause your body to produce serotonin. If you can stimulate serotonin production through exercise, you should not crave high-calorie carbohydrate foods as much.

4. Exercise renews your spirit.

Mindful exercise allows you a "time out" from life during which you can rekindle your energy and renew your spirit. Your exercise time will be "your" time, a time of freedom from life's responsibilities, obligations, and worries. It will no longer be a drudgery for you. That is because during mindful exercise you will have a completely different attitude than you've ever had toward exercise before.

··

MINDFUL EXERCISE: AFTER-MEAL WALKING AND THE SPIRIT OF RENEWAL

What do I mean by mindful exercise? How does mindful exercise differ from any other kind of exercise? Is mindful exercise walking, swimming, aerobics, bicycling, weight lifting? The answer is that it is all of these. It is not a type of exercise but an attitude you have while you are exercising.

Keep in mind that mindfulness as applied to exercise or anything else consists of four elements:

1. Paying attention
2. Increasing awareness
3. Focusing only on the present moment
4. Being an observer, not a judge

My mindful exercise plan consists of:

- Walking with a mindful attitude
- For a duration of 20 to 30 minutes
- After two meals or snacks a day

What I want you to do is walk after any two meals or snacks a day. Your walk should last 20 to 30 minutes. You can walk fast or slow, depending on how you feel. The important thing is that you walk with a mindful attitude.

The most important thing about exercising or walking with a mindful attitude is that you focus on the present moment. As you walk (whether it is outdoors in your neighborhood or indoors on a treadmill), the past and future should not exist for you. You should focus on the present moment. You should not be thinking about what happened over the past few minutes or hours or what is going to happen when you are finished exercising. You should not be planning your schedule or making a list of the things you need to be doing. You must be mindful. You must be paying attention and being aware of the present moment.

The present moment includes what you are seeing, hearing, touching, or smelling. It includes what you are feeling. It includes thoughts, emotions, and physical sensations. It does *not* include what has just happened or what is about to happen.

Neither does your mindful exercise time include judgments. You might be aware of your body and your feelings. You are not to judge or evaluate. If you hear yourself saying, "This is boring. I hate exercise. It's not fair that I have to do this," realize that this is an evaluation, not an observation. The observer would simply be aware of this thought and let it go.

A mindful exerciser does not worry about how fast or how far he or she is going. If you are being mindful, you do not think, "I wonder how much longer I need to go," or "I have walked 20 minutes, I only have 10 minutes to go." If you have these thoughts, observe them and be aware of them but do not get caught up in them. Your attitude should be, "It is interesting that I am so worried about how much longer I have to go." You are an outside observer looking in at yourself. You are not involved. You are objective and impartial.

When you adopt this mindful attitude, your exercise will go very quickly. It will not feel like a chore. When you are mindful, time is fleeting. Your walk will seem to pass in a moment. But in the process of your exercise, you will learn a great deal about your mind and body. It will be an opportunity for you.

It is important for you to view your after-meal walk as "your" time. It is your time for renewal. You are *choosing* to walk. You do not *have* to exercise, it is always your choice. Your after-meal walk is your special time. It is your time away from life. It is your time to renew your mind, body, and spirit. No one can take this time away from you and you should not allow anyone to take it away from you.

....

WHY WALK AFTER MEALS?

After-meal walking is important for two reasons. First, it makes a definite end to a meal or snack. It signifies that eating is over and another activity is about to begin. It provides an incompatible alternative to continued eating. It helps you avoid overeating. You eat and then you burn those calories by walking. This is not excessive compensation, it simply demonstrates to you on a daily basis the association between input and output.

Second, after-meal walking is valuable because it burns more calories than walking at any other time of the day. This is due to thermogenesis. Thermogenesis is a process by which your metabolism burns extra calories in response to a meal or snack.

After eating, your body must work harder to digest, break down, and assimilate the nutrients that you just ate. This process requires your body to work harder, to burn more calories. In fact, your metabolism increases 15 to 20 percent after each meal and remains increased for one to three hours. When you walk after a meal or snack while thermogenesis is occurring, you burn even more calories. The blending of thermogenesis and walking supercharges your metabolism and causes it to burn maximum calories. The result is a multiple effect so that you are burning more calories with 20 to 30 minutes of walking after eating than you would if you were to walk at any other time of the day.

WHAT'S MORE IMPORTANT, TIME OR DISTANCE?

I want you to concentrate on exercising 20 to 30 minutes after two meals a day. Time is more important than distance. Studies show that you will be more consistent with your exercise program if you focus on time, not distance. In this way, if you feel sluggish and tired, you can take your time. Just put in your 20 minutes. On days when you feel more vigorous and energetic, let it all out and walk faster, traveling a greater distance. Just remember that time is the key. Twenty or thirty minutes after two meals or snacks is your goal.

SCHEDULING YOUR WALKS

Just as it is very important to schedule specific times for meals and snacks each day (refer to Chapter 11), it is essential that your after-meal walks be scheduled.

New habits are built on routine and repetition. You must set up a schedule and stick to it.

You may choose to walk after any two meals or snacks a day. For instance, you might walk after breakfast and lunch or after breakfast and your mid-afternoon snack. It doesn't matter as long as you block that time out of your schedule so nothing else can interfere with your walk. Some people keep their walking routine the same, day after day. Others modify it on weekends. If you have a busy, hectic schedule you may change each day. You must, however, plan at the beginning of each day exactly when you will be taking your two walks that day.

HOW TO HANDLE PERFECTIONISM

The most important aspect of your exercise program is consistency. The weight-control competition is a tortoise and hare race and the slow and steady tortoise always wins. You must be careful of your tendency to be all-or-nothing. When you first begin this program, you will be tempted to do more exercise than I am asking you to do. At your first slip, you may want to give up your exercise altogether. This is your old pattern and you must change it.

One way to deal with perfectionism with regard to exercise is to set your standards lower, not higher. Dr. David Burns, a psychiatrist on the faculty of the

University of Pennsylvania School of Medicine, specializes in teaching people how to change their perfectionistic thinking patterns. He tells the story about how he applied his teachings to his personal exercise program. When Dr. Burns began jogging several years ago he could not run more than two or three hundred yards without giving up. Under these circumstances, the perfectionist would try harder, pushing himself or herself to the limit. No measure of success would be good enough, since perfection is impossible.

Dr. Burns made it his aim to run a little less far each day than he did the day before. The result was that he could accomplish his goal easily. This would make him feel so good that he would jog farther, far more than his goal for the day. Using this method of not trying as hard, Dr. Burns built himself up to the point that he was jogging seven miles a day. He swears by this approach for perfectionists and advises them to "dare to aim at being average."

I know at first blush this method sounds counterproductive, but believe me it works. I have seen it work with hundreds of clients. As a perfectionist, you can even demonstrate willpower by taking an occasional day off from your exercise, not on a day when you don't feel like exercising, but on a day when you can't wait to get out there for your walk.

....

WHAT ABOUT OTHER EXERCISES BESIDES WALKING?

I believe that walking is the very best exercise. However, if you choose to bicycle, swim, or do aerobics, that is perfectly all right. Just remember to approach these exercises with a mindful attitude.

After you break your binge-eating pattern and begin to lose weight, I would like you to add resistance training to your exercise regimen. Resistance training is weight lifting. I suggest this because of two reasons. First, resistance training increases muscle tissue in your body. Since muscle is very chemically active even at rest, it increases your metabolism. In fact, the more muscle in your body, the higher your metabolism. Second, resistance training tones your muscles, which improves your body image.

When you reach this point in your program, I strongly advise you to join a local health club. Clients of mine who try to do resistance training on their own usually have trouble sticking with it. At a fitness facility, you have professional instruction, the right equipment, and others around you who are doing the same thing. In addition to daily walking, my wife, Gabrielle, and I work out three times a week at a fitness club. In this way, we encourage each other and share a common interest.

....

A NOTE OF CAUTION

This mindful exercise program involves moderate exercise and is designed for overweight individuals who are relatively healthy. If you have special medical problems such as heart trouble, high blood pressure, respiratory problems, or recurrent back pain, check with your physician before starting. Walking should be done at a moderate pace. If you are breathing so hard that you cannot carry on a normal conversation, you are overdoing it.

CHAPTER 18

....

Holidays and Other High-Risk Situations

Some food situations are more difficult to deal with than others. The most successful binge eaters learn to identify which specific circumstances cause the most temptation for them. Then, they develop a plan of action on how to deal with high-risk situations.

A high-risk situation is any set of circumstances that puts you more at risk for binge eating. It could be a holiday when tempting food is available and leftovers are plentiful. It might be a situation in which you are alone and upset. You must think about and identify your top five high-risk situations and develop a detailed plan to deal with them.

The important key is to plan ahead. Do not wait for these circumstances to occur before you figure out what to do. Willpower is not just a matter of toughing it out. It is being mindful, being aware, and planning for action.

Preparing ahead of time for high-risk food situations is even more important for overweight binge eaters than for overweight people who do not binge. Studies show that to overcome your binge eating and to avoid a relapse you must be very aware of situations that can overwhelm you. You must be careful of being too sure of yourself. You must be confident and determined but you also must remain vigilant.

When I discussed mindful willpower in Chapter 10 I spoke of the need for mindful awareness. I advised you to become more aware of your eating and everything associated with it. This heightened awareness must continue as a regular part of your life, even after your binge eating stops. I am not talking about obsession and I certainly do not want you to become a fanatic about diet and nutrition, but you should realize that this is something you'll have to deal with for the rest of your life.

....

WEEKLY PLANNING SESSION

To stay vigilant about high-risk situations, schedule a planning session once a week. This should be a regularly scheduled time such as prior to bedtime on Sunday evening or first thing on Monday morning. During this time, think ahead over the next week and identify any situations, no matter how small, that may interfere with your progress. What circumstances might upset you, tempt you to eat, or keep you from exercising? Are any holiday celebrations coming up? Will your life be more stressful next week? Will you be busier? Are there any dinner parties that may tempt you? Will you be entertaining and have more food in your house than usual? Are you traveling for business or pleasure? Will you be alone more often next week? These situations will not automatically trigger a binge but they put you at a greater risk for one.

Take time to write down next week's high-risk situations. This planning session should be part of your routine each and every week. Do not discontinue this habit just because you haven't binged in a while. I have seen clients make this mistake and then they are blindsided by a high-risk temptation that they should have been aware of and could have planned for.

PLANNING FOR SUCCESS

Once you have identified each week's high-risk situations, it is time to develop a specific plan of action to deal with each. Your plan should be broken down into what you will do to help you cope *before*, *during*, and *after* the situation occurs. It is helpful to put this plan into written form so that, after the fact, you can review whether or not you implemented all aspects of it.

I'll show you how to plan in this way using a holiday celebration as an example, a high-risk situation that is often troublesome for binge eaters.

....

OVERCOMING HOLIDAY
TEMPTATIONS

Holidays can be a particularly risky time for binge eaters. Certainly, there is a lot of extra food around and more high-fat, high-calorie food than is normally available. There exists an expectation that you will eat more than usual. It is one of the few times when people give themselves and everyone else permission to eat.

Holiday traditions keep us bound to old eating habits. You must begin to challenge those traditions. You should not deprive yourself on holidays but you should make healthier changes in the way you and your family celebrate. To give you an example of how to go about planning for a holiday celebration, let's take Thanksgiving as an example.

Start by thinking about what you might do to prepare yourself *before* Thanksgiving arrives. Here are some preplanning strategies.

1. Question your traditions and take the opportunity to begin new ones that will help you avoid binge eating. You could arrange to do something totally different for Thanksgiving. Instead of a family food fest, plan to take a trip or a special excursion for the holiday. This might be a time to "expand your horizons" as I mentioned in Chapter 16 as part of your new self-image. Go on a ski trip, head

to the beach, or drive to the mountains. You might decide to practice the real meaning of the holiday by doing volunteer work to help others.

2. Make a list of the reasons why you want to overcome your binge-eating problem. Give thought to how life will be different when you defeat binge eating and lose weight.

3. Close your eyes and imagine yourself during the holiday celebration. Visualize yourself making positive, portion-controlled food choices and feeling good about what you are doing.

4. If you are bringing a dish to the holiday meal, consider making a lower-calorie, lower-fat item. If you are hosting the celebration, prepare a variety of alternatives, some lower in calories and some not, to make choices easier for you as well as for the other guests.

5. If you are preparing the meal, prepare less than usual. Most people cook too much food for holiday celebrations and then have to contend with leftovers. Give leftovers to family members to take home with them.

6. Take into consideration that holidays, although joyous events, can be associated with emotional distress. Family get-togethers can stimulate old conflicts. Holidays can also trigger emotional stress by reminding you of better times or of relatives or friends who are no longer with you. Take time to prepare yourself by practicing the five ways to gain control over your emotions that I described in Chapter 13.

7. If you spend your holidays doing for others and trying to please everyone, remember what I told you in Chapter 14 about taking care of yourself. Always schedule some "you" time during the holidays to nurture yourself.

8. Do not skip meals during the day of the holiday meal. Stick with the six eating times a day that I recommend. You want to avoid hunger.

9. You must stay mindful and aware of your eating even at holiday time. One recent study showed that a group of people who kept daily written records of everything they were eating between Thanksgiving and New Year's *lost* an average of seven pounds during this time. Most people gain this amount of weight over the holidays.

These are planning strategies to consider *during* the event.

1. Decide whether or not to drink alcohol. Alcohol can lower your resolve and trigger overeating. If you do drink, make sure you decide ahead of time what and how much you will be drinking. Limit yourself to one glass of wine with the meal, for example.

2. During the holiday celebration, focus your attention on the people, not the food. Involve yourself in conversations. Practice people-mindfulness by paying particular attention to what people look like, how they are dressed, and what they are saying.

3. Be careful of feelings of deprivation, the "poor me" syndrome. Watch your self-talk. Stop during the get-together to challenge negative thinking such as "Everyone else seems to be having such a good time, eating and drinking whatever they like. I wish I could be like them." You might dispute this thought with, "I feel good about my self-restraint. I feel strong and in control. It's too bad everyone else can't be as determined as I feel today."

4. Don't deprive yourself. Keep in mind that food is not the enemy and that you are no longer a slave to all-or-nothing thinking or all-or-nothing eating. Control your eating with portion control. Take the pumpkin pie if you wish but just have a small-to-moderate-size serving.

5. Eat slowly and mindfully. Enjoy your meal and pay attention to how the food looks and tastes. Practice mindful awareness. Pay attention to your feelings of fullness. Try to be one of the last people at the table to finish your meal (even if others choose to have seconds).

6. Pay no attention to "friendly enemies" who encourage you to overindulge. Respond with a polite, but firm, "no thank you." Do not use dieting as a reason for refusing offers of food. You are no longer a dieter.

7. Take a walk after the meal. Encourage others to join you, but if they don't, do your own thing and go by yourself.

8. If you slip up and overeat, watch your "all-or-

nothing" thinking. Forgive yourself and return to your original plan. You are not perfect, and you don't have to be.

Finally, you must devise a plan for *after* Thanksgiving.

1. If you are alone after the celebration is over, this may be a higher-risk time than the holiday mealtime itself. Plan not to have leftovers readily available, go to bed early, or stay close to someone else to help you keep from bingeing.
2. If you slipped up and ate more than you had planned, do not allow negative, all-or-nothing thinking to get the best of you. Challenge these thoughts as I taught you in Chapter 14.
3. Take time to evaluate your plan. How did it work out? Pay particular attention to your successes. Practice mindful willpower as I discussed in Chapter 10 by paying attention to the thoughts and feelings that you used when you were tempted and did not succumb. Write the secrets of your success in your Willpower Journal.

A FINAL WORD ABOUT PLANNING

Weekly planning is very important for your success. Binge eaters who plan in this way are much more successful than those who do not. The secret is in scheduling your planning session once a week and sticking to this schedule. Once you identify upcoming high-risk situations, make sure your plan is very specific. In fact, the more detailed it is the better. As you progress, this planning will take less and less time because you will be learning to handle more and more difficult food situations.

CHAPTER 19

······························

Relapse Prevention: Progress, Not Perfection

Once you have conquered your binge eating and have lost weight, I am certain that your dream is to avoid binge eating completely for the rest of your life. Realistically speaking, many binge eaters have occasional lapses in their eating behavior. These lapses are few and far between and they should not bother you. They are so infrequent that they should not even affect your weight. It is important for you to deal with them in a mindful way so that you do not fall back into your old all-or-nothing thinking. A lapse is simply a temporary setback.

A relapse, on the other hand, occurs when lapses continue, you lose awareness, and you fall back into your former binge patterns. The key to preventing a relapse is mindful awareness. You must remain continually aware of your behavior by establishing a system of accountability.

You must continue to put into practice all of the mental, emotional, and behavioral changes that comprise the Mindful-Eating Program. It is not enough to stop binge eating and lose weight. The changes you have made with this program are permanent. They are meant not only to help you overcome binge eating and lose weight but also to improve your happiness and well-being. You should view them as life skills that you need to stay in control.

As your binge eating improves, you may have a tendency to become complacent about the changes you have made. When this happens, you may gradually "forget" to implement some of the program components or think you don't need them anymore. This is dangerous thinking that leads to a gradual erosion of the Mindful-Eating Program. Then, under conditions of stress or extreme temptation, you may binge and fall back into your old ways.

The best way to stay aware and to maintain your vigilance is to review your progress once a week. You should schedule this review when you weigh yourself or when you are planning for high-risk situations (as discussed in Chapter 18). When I refer to progress I am talking about the *process* of your success not the *outcome*. That is, you may tell me you have been very successful because you have not binged in a month and you have lost 15 pounds. This is a successful outcome. However, if the process is not successfully intact, if you are not eating mindfully six times a day or practicing the Body Scan to improve your self-image, you are asking for trouble. These new behaviors and new ways of looking at yourself and your eating are the underpinnings of the program. These changes must be maintained no matter what.

....

THE MINDFUL-EATING
PROGRAM WEEKLY REVIEW

When you review your progress once a week I want you to take the Mindful-Eating Program Review test. This is a 20-item test I have devised to help you take an inventory of how you are doing. It also reminds you of all the components of the program and helps you stay accountable for doing them.

THE MINDFUL-EATING PROGRAM REVIEW

For each of the following questions, give yourself:

    3 points for each *Always* answer
    2 points for each *Usually* answer
    1 point for each *Sometimes* answer
    0 points for each *Rarely* or *Never* answer

1. Are you eating three meals and three snacks a day?
2. Are you eating on a planned schedule?
3. Are you eating without distractions from other activities?
4. Are you controlling portion sizes?
5. Are you scheduling serving-size binge foods into your eating plans?

6. Are you leaving one morsel of food on your plate to demonstrate your power over food?

7. While eating, are you practicing a mindful-eating style?

8. Are you practicing the Quiet Meal?

9. Are you paying attention to hunger and satiety before and during meals and snacks?

10. Are you being mindful of the secrets of your success by keeping a Willpower Journal?

11. Are you using my five ways to achieve emotional freedom (increasing awareness of emotions, releasing or quieting emotions, confronting emotions, solving problems that cause emotions, letting emotions go)?

12. Are you practicing mindful thinking awareness by regularly examining your negative, all-or-nothing thoughts?

13. Are you writing down your negative thoughts when they occur, challenging their logic and writing a new mental script for you to follow?

14. Are you practicing the Body Scan to help you develop a better awareness and acceptance of your body weight and shape?

15. Are you confronting your mirror image to improve body image?

16. Are you practicing the Self Scan to improve your self-esteem?

17. Are you being true to yourself and expressing how you really think and feel to others?

18. Are you balancing your "Wants" and "Shoulds" and dreaming your dreams?

19. Are you taking two scheduled after-meal walks a day?
20. Are you regularly identifying high-risk situations and developing plans to deal with them?

After you complete your answers, score the test using the scoring system on this page. Here's how to interpret your score:

Total Score

45–60	**Excellent**—keep up the good work
30–44	**Good**—you are doing well but you could be more consistent
15–29	**Caution**—you are in the borderline range and should try to improve
0–14	**Danger**—you are falling back into your old habits and are risking a relapse

You should take this test and score it each and every week. If you are doing well, this is good reinforcement and feedback for you. If you are having trouble, reread those chapters that pertain to the areas that are causing you the most difficulty. If you are in the *Danger* zone you might want to reread the entire book and go back to basics. Don't think of yourself as a failure. You may be dealing with difficult life situations that are causing you more stress than usual. Your time may not be your own lately and you are losing track of taking proper care of yourself. The important thing is to nip these warning signs in the bud. That's why the Mindful-Eating Program Review test is so essential to your continued progress. Take it every week without fail.

....

WHEN TO CALL IN THE PROFESSIONALS

If you find that you are having difficulty with repeated relapses you may need professional help. You may be suffering from more severe problems such as clinical depression, which may be hindering your progress. Under these circumstances I would suggest you consult a health professional who is familiar with binge-eating disorder. These specialists are usually psychologists who treat obesity, binge eating, and/or eating disorders. Ask your physician for a referral or check the telephone Yellow Pages for a specialist. A nearby medical school or university may have a binge-eating program or a weight-management program that treats this problem.

A traditional diet program will not help you. You need very special help. Basically, you need a professional who is familiar with the type of program I have outlined and who can help you implement it.

CHAPTER 20

······························

A Final Word

As my final word, I want to wish you well with your new binge-free life. If you follow *Binge Breaker!*, you will be able to overcome your binge eating and you will finally be able to make progress in losing weight. I have seen people who have been binge eaters for years finally conquer their problem and all the guilt, discouragement, and depression that accompany it.

I don't care how many times you have tried to lose weight in the past and failed. You have learned that binge eating has been your downfall. You are not weak-willed. You have not been a failure. You were simply approaching the problem of weight loss in the wrong way. Your problem was binge eating, not lack of motivation or determination.

I hear so many of my clients talk about themselves as if they were a different breed. They think of themselves as weak and addicted. Many of them have given up. I have seen the most discouraged of them find a new spirit of renewal, take charge of life, put an end to binge eating, and lose weight. Most important, life has become a totally new experience for them. They are no longer dependent on food. They feel free for the first time in their lives.

I want my book to represent hope to you. I want you to feel that someone finally understands your problem. The program I have outlined can work for you. I have seen it work time and time again, even among those who, because of their past failures at losing weight, were skeptical at first.

Just remember that the key is mindfulness not only as it applies to food but also to your life in general. Mindfulness will help you change your relationship to food once and for all. It will help you improve your self-image and how you feel about yourself. It will set you free.

Enjoy your new freedom—and your new life.

Index

Index

INDEX

About the Author

PETER M. MILLER, Ph.D., founded the Hilton Head Health Institute on Hilton Head Island, South Carolina, in 1976. Dr. Miller received a bachelor of arts degree from the University of Maryland and a doctorate in clinical psychology from the University of South Carolina. He holds a faculty appointment in the Department of Health Promotion and Education at the University of South Carolina. He is the author of 11 books, 70 research articles, and is editor in chief of the scientific journal *Addictive Behaviors*. Dr. Miller's work has been profiled on television as well as in national magazines.